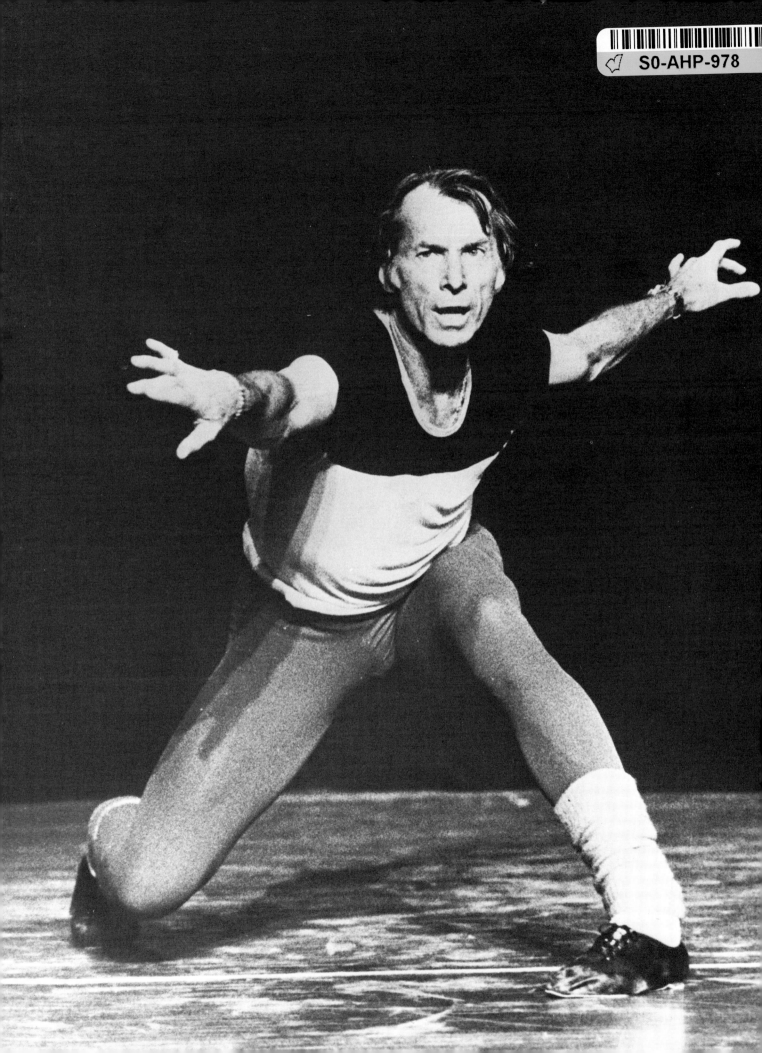

Dedicated to Matt Mattox and Jorunn Kirkenær for showing me the way to a unique art form—JAZZ ART.

The Matt Mattox Book of Jazz Dance

Elisabeth Frich

Foreword and Comments by Matt Mattox

STERLING PUBLISHING CO., INC.   NEW YORK
Distributed in the U.K. by Blandford Press

Other Books of Interest
Dancer's Audition Book
Dancing as a Career for Men
Jazz Dance

Dancers pictured in the book:
Matt Mattox
Annette Plottin
Kari Helgesen
Arne Norum
Elisabeth Frich

Library of Congress Cataloging in Publication Data

Frich, Elisabeth.
 The Matt Mattox book of jazz dance.

 Includes index.
 1. Jazz dance. I. Mattox, Matt. II. Title.
GV1753.F75 1983   793.3   83-4647
ISBN 0-8069-7048-0
ISBN 0-8069-7662-4 (pbk.)

Copyright © 1983 by Sterling Publishing Co., Inc.
Two Park Avenue, New York, N.Y. 10016
Distributed in Australia by Oak Tree Press Co., Ltd.
P.O. Box K514 Haymarket, Sydney 2000, N.S.W.
Distributed in the United Kingdom by Blandford Press
Link House, West Street, Poole, Dorset BH15 1LL, England
Distributed in Canada by Oak Tree Press Ltd.
% Canadian Manda Group, P.O. Box 920, Station U
Toronto, Ontario, Canada M8Z 5P9
Manufactured in the United States of America
All rights reserved

Contents

Note: Matt Mattox' comments appear on the exercise pages, followed by his initials.

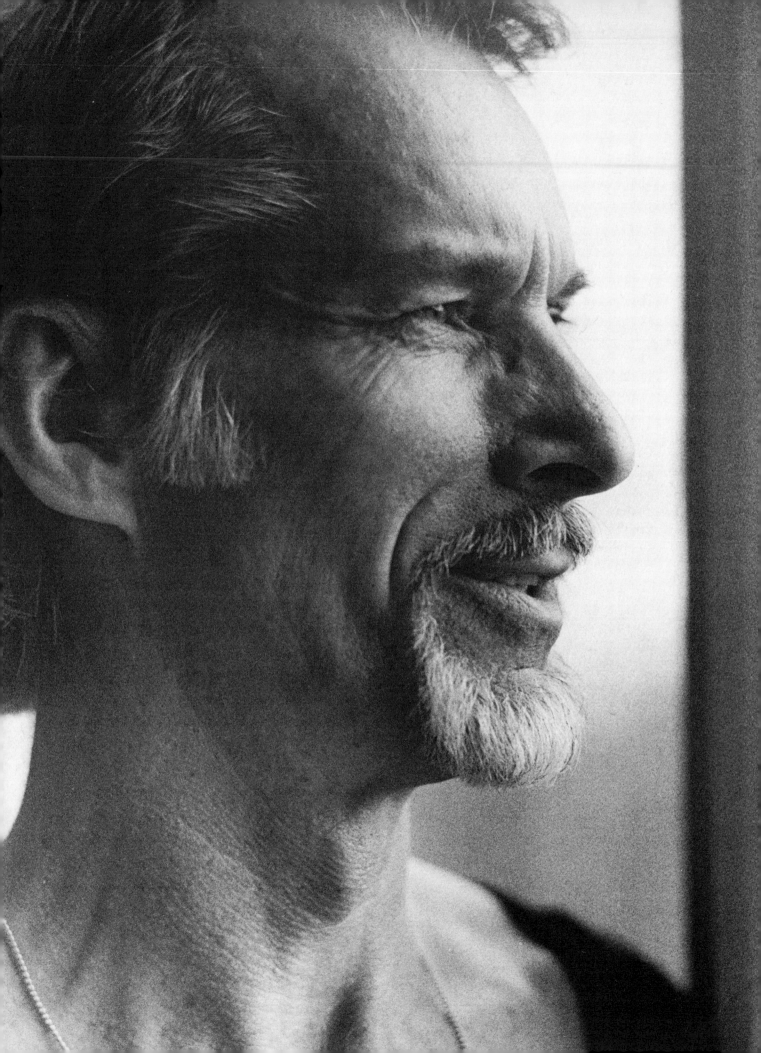

Foreword by Matt Mattox

The warm-ups and isolation exercises in this book embody my particular system of teaching "modern jazz" dance. Elisabeth Frich, a student to be proud of and herself a performer and teacher, has diligently compiled all of the information and photos for this book. Not only is she a beautiful student and dancer, but she is an untiring worker and an enthusiast of my work. With her dedication and perseverance in pulling this material together, she has fulfilled a task that I, myself, have never found the time to do.

The volume that she has created is a reference book that can be used on many levels by an entire spectrum of dancers and students, whether or not they have worked with the exercises before—whether or not they have danced before. Of course, beginners, looking at this book, won't be able to achieve as much as they might if they were to come to class every day—or even two or three times a week. But any student, studying the photos and captions and practicing the exercises daily, will eventually become aware of the rhythm of the exercises and the benefits to be derived from them. And even if students simply practice the exercises a few times a week, they will discover for themselves the advantages they offer in helping to build a healthy, well-conditioned body. For students who have never studied dance before, this toning and conditioning could be an important reward.

Dancers will find even more benefits here. For the dancer who has studied only one technique, the exercises will re-awaken their comprehension of the placement of the body, from a different point of view.

Many professional dancers—after weeks of training in these and other exercises—have told me that they have discovered new things about their own technique which they had never thought of before.

Concentrating on working individual parts of the body, for example—from the point of view of isolation—creates a new kind of liaison between body and brain, which may never have been sensed before.

The exercises may create a new awareness of the sensations taking place in the body at any given moment. Many dancers today do not seem to work from the point of view of sensations, and this consciousness is valuable to every dancer.

But even more important, in my opinion, are the benefits these exercises provide from the standpoint of coordination. Developing coordination as a dancer doesn't just happen. It may take years to work through, but when the metamorphosis is complete, the dancer has undergone a remarkable transformation. These exercises, concentrating as they do on coordination, will hasten that glorious change.

For the choreographer, too, these exercises will be enormously useful. Often, one's mind gets tired of creating. If it is essential that you continue to create, you can use the isolations shown here to refresh those creative energies as they reveal how to use the body from a completely different point of view. I've been using them—with changes, of course, additions and deletions—over a period of 24 years, and I have always found them to be a stimulant to my creativity.

Research is important to anyone who is creative, but research without a basic system to work from is of no importance. All the isolations in this form of dance (these exercises are only a part of them) can be of the greatest value to creative choreography.

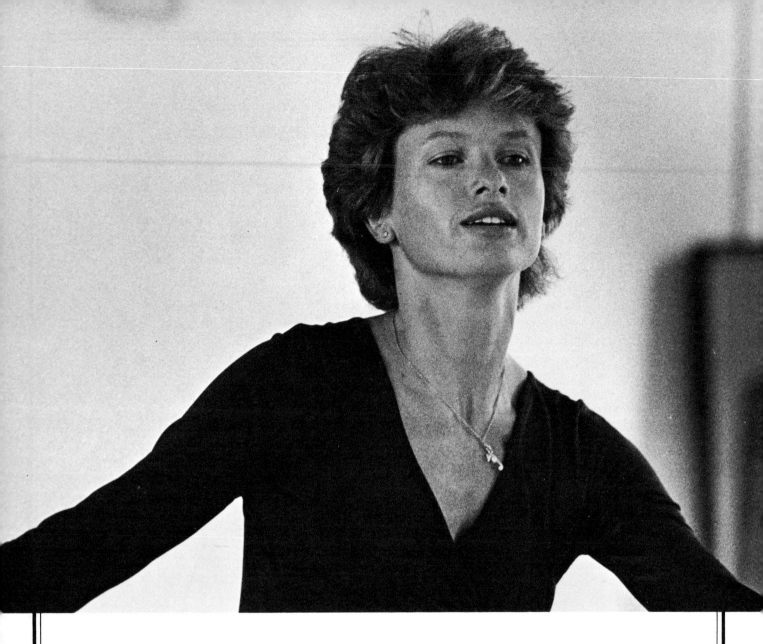

Acknowledgments

I would like to thank Jan Fredrik Larsen for all his work with the instructional photos and for never losing faith in this project. My warm thanks also to the other photographers for their contributions to this book.

I am very grateful for the beautiful work and patience of Annette Plottin, Kari Helgesen, Arne Norum and Matt Mattox who have given endless hours of their valuable time modelling for the photographs.

This book could never have been brought about without the support and inspiration of my students and colleagues and the encouragement of my teacher Jorunn Kirkenær, the director of Den Norske Balletthøyskole in Oslo. She introduced Matt Mattox in Norway and started me off on this project. I thank her for giving me the opportunity to research and specialize in this unique jazz art technique.

My deepest gratitude to Matt Mattox, for trusting in me to write this book, and for his guidance along the way. I hope I have managed to convey some of his spirit in this book—the spirit of a warm personality, an excellent teacher and a creative choreographer.

Introduction

This book is the result of many years of training, performing and teaching jazz dance, dating back to the summer of 1970, when I finished my full-time study at "Den Norske Balletthøyskole." Matt Mattox was invited by my teacher Jorunn Kirkenær to teach at a course in Oslo. For two weeks we struggled like crazy just to be able to *follow* the intricate movements and the high speed of this dynamic teacher. I thought I would never ever be able to *dance* it.

But my curiosity about this unique style had been awakened, and after two years of studying Mattox' jazz art technique thoroughly in London, I returned to Norway knowing I had been given a gift which would be valuable to me for a lifetime of work in dance: a *system* for training and teaching jazz and a great source of inspiration for choreography.

I began teaching at "Den Norske Balletthøyskole," and soon felt the need for written material for my students about jazz training. That's what got me started on this project, but I quickly realized that I ought to share my knowledge with many more students, dancers and teachers. I hope this system will inspire you—from the first plié to the last jump—the way it has inspired me and so many others.

Now—just a few bits of information about how to use this book. We've tried to show every important move in the photos. In a few cases, some of the dancers have been turned a bit in order to make the movement clearer. But if you follow the space diagram on page 11, you'll be able to keep the sequence going in the right direction.

It's up to you how many times you do each exercise—and it depends on what you (or your students) need. A general rule is to start with pliés, tendus and some leg exercises before going to the isolations: head, shoulders, ribcage and pelvis. Some stretches, especially for the back of the legs, are always done before the kicks and jumps. After some good stretching and strengthening exercises on the floor, you should be ready to put it all into—DANCE!

If you find some of the series long and complicated, pick out what you can do, leave out some of the arm-work to begin with, and slowly build up to the whole exercise. When you know them well, you can start "playing around" by combining the exercises in different ways: Take one part of a shoulder isolation and add on part of *another* shoulder isolation, for instance. In this way, you have a system you can stick to, but you won't get bored, because your brain has to stay awake to new variations. Also, you get warmed up very quickly if you combine several exercises into one long series without stopping.

For accompaniment, use any type of jazz and modern music, as long as it has a steady beat, mostly in 4/4 rhythm. Try to challenge your body to do the exercises in quick tempo at the end!

Good luck! And remember: "JAZZ IS JOY!"

Elisabeth Frich
Oslo, Norway
April, 1983

Note: A video cassette of Matt Mattox' "Jazz Art Technique," demonstrated by the master himself together with Annette Plottin, includes 45 of his favorite warm-up exercises and a long dance routine. The 45-minute cassette is supplementary to this book and is available on VHS, Betamax, U-matic, VCR and VCR 1500 and 1700 systems. It may be ordered from:

Jazz Art Productions
Elisabeth Frich
P.O. Box 5144
Majorstua,
Oslo 3, Norway
Phone: (02) 60.38.10

Photographs: on page 1, credit F. Levieux. On pages 6, 13, 48 and 75, credit Lesley Leslie-Spinks. On pages 8, 27 and 51, credit Inge Fjelldalen. On pages 59 and 85, credit Olav Hasselknippe. On page 103, credit J.P. Lelièvre. On pages 106 to 113, credit Norman Henderson.

Positions of Feet

ABBREVIATIONS:

C—Center
L—Left
R—Right
p—position
pp—parallel position
pt—point (see space diagram, right, below)

FIRST POSITION

1p turned out— 1pp— 1p turned in

SECOND POSITION

2p turned out—

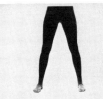

2pp—   2p turned in

FOURTH POSITION

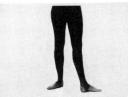 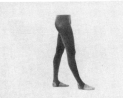

4 p turned out (open: a   4pp (distance between feet
straight line from heel to   equivalent to 1pp)
heel)

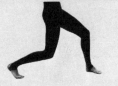

4p turned in (front leg turned in, back leg parallel)

Third and fifth positions are seldom used in this style.

Positions on Floor

FIRST POSITION

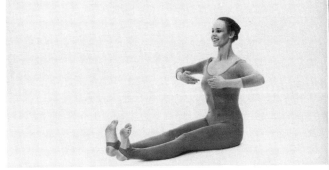

1pp (with arms in 1p also)

SECOND POSITION

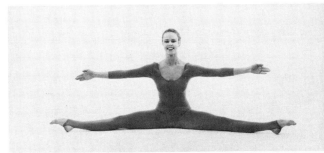

2p turned out (arms in 2p)

FOURTH POSITION

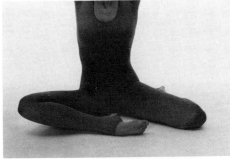

4p: Sit on both hips with back leg pulled in to the hip. Keep legs very open, knees in a straight line.

Space Diagram

BACK

```
        5
  4 ┌ ─ ─ ┼ ─ ─ ┐ 6
    │  ╲     ╱   │
RIGHT 3 ┼ ─ ( ) ─ ┼ 7 LEFT
    │  ╱     ╲   │
  2 └ ─ ─ ┼ ─ ─ ┘ 8
        1
```

FRONT

11

ARMS DOWN

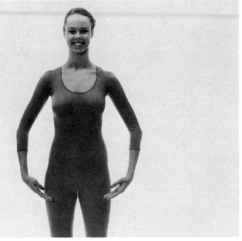

The arms are rounded and held slightly out from the thighs.

FIRST POSITION

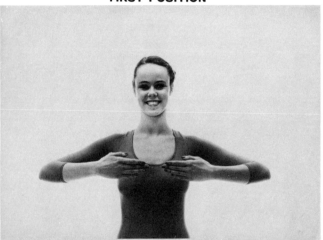

Arms are bent in front of the chest with elbows lifted to the side and palms in. Keep space between upper arms and chest.

SECOND POSITION

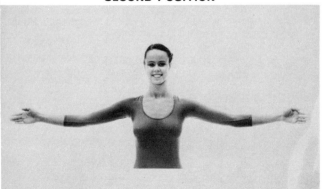

Arms are stretched to the side (palms forward) slightly below shoulder level and in front of the body. In some isolation exercises, elbows may be bent more, and in combinations they may be stretched more ("reach to infinity").

THIRD POSITION

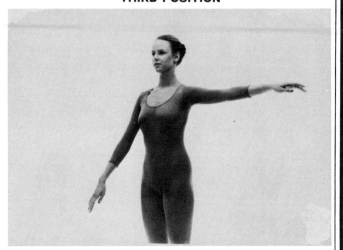

LOW—1 arm in 2p (palm down)
1 arm down (palm in)

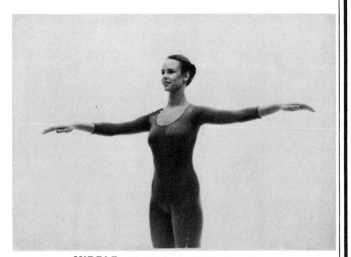

MIDDLE—1 arm in 2p (palm down)
1 arm forward (palm down)

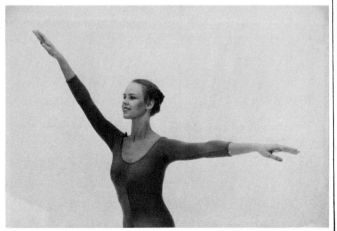

HIGH—1 arm in 2p (palm down)
1 arm up (palm forward and slightly out)

See page 122 for definitions of terms used in this book.

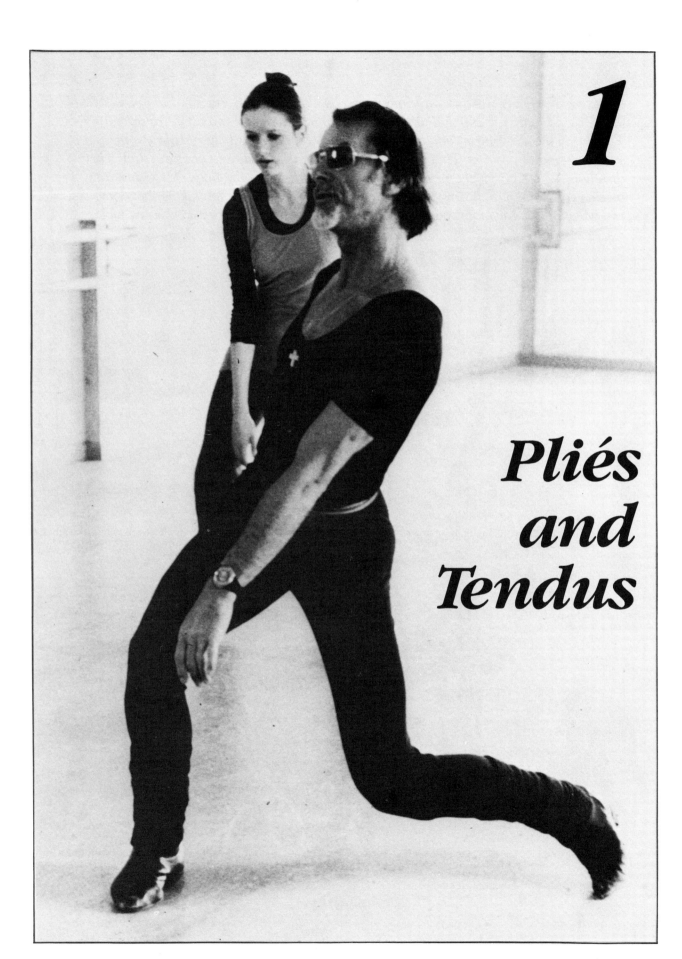

1

*Pliés
and
Tendus*

In the classical dance we work with 5 positions: 1st, 2nd, 3rd, 4th and 5th, but in this style of dance we use only 1st, 2nd and 4th. The pliés which follow are important in several ways. They begin the warm-up of your hip, knee and ankle joints. They help you place your body in a correct standing position. They make you aware of the idea that your body can stretch in two directions—up towards the ceiling as well as down towards the floor. They start you off placing your arms and moving them in decided patterns. And as you follow the sequences, you will also become more conscious of using the long stretched leg and pointed foot.

—MM.

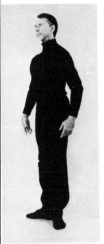 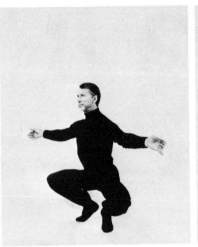 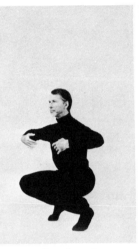 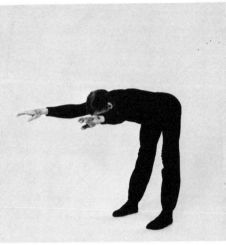

PART 1
START in 1p, turned out with arms down.

1-4 Grand plié with arms to 2p. Start arms with accent; then continue softly.

AND close legs to pp. Bring arms to 1p.

5-8 Stretch forward with a straight back. Stretch arms forward parallel to floor, palms down.

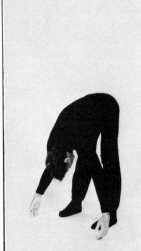 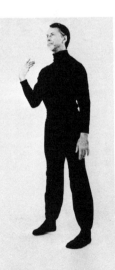 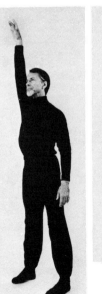 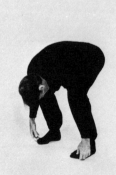

1-2 Drop upper body and arms.
3-4 Roll up through spine to standing

position. Fold R arm on the way and stretch it up, palm forward.

5   Fold R arm and release down. Sway back and let upper body fall. Lift head back.

6   Finish release with rounded back and arms, head relaxed. Head comes last. Throw it down with force.

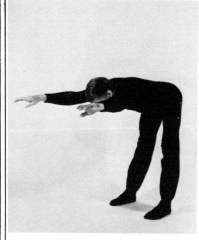

7-8 Stretch forward with straight back at 90° angle. Stretch arms forward parallel to floor, palms down.

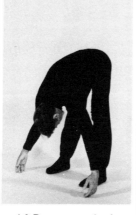

1-2 Drop upper body and arms.

3-4 Fold arms and stretch them up.

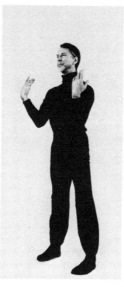

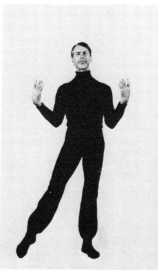

5-6 Release

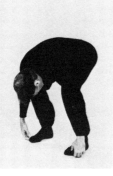

and down with both arms.

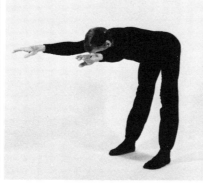

7-8 Stretch forward with straight back at 90° angle. Stretch arms forward parallel to floor, palms down.

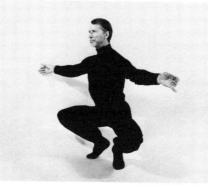

AND 1 Turn out and sit in grand plié with upper body C. Arms go through 1p to 2p.

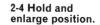

2-4 Hold and enlarge position.

5-6 Straighten knees and lower heels.

7 Lower arms.

8 Turn feet to pp, weight, weight forward.

ON TO PART **2**

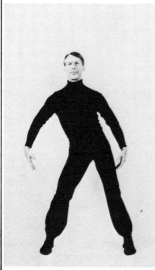

PART 2

1 Place R leg bent in 2pp. Contract L side. Lift L hip diagonally up.

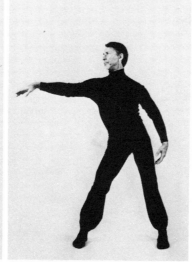

2-8 Stretch R arm to 2p while softly deepening contraction on L side. Look out over R arm.

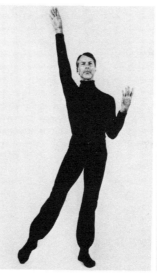

1-2 Push weight to L leg with R leg stretched to side parallel. Stretch R arm up, palm forward. Fold L arm. Accent.

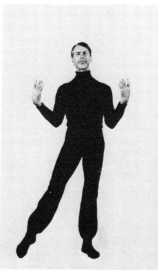

3-4 Fold R arm.

1. Pliés in 1st and 2nd Position (page 3)

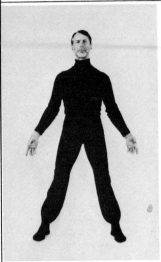 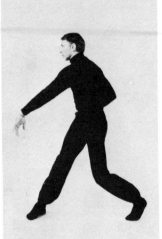 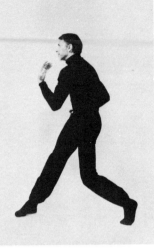 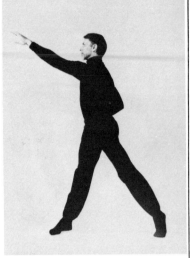

5-8 Softly lower R heel with equal weight on both legs in 2pp. Stretch arms diagonally down, palms forward.

1 Contract R side and turn shoulders to R by lifting up into diaphragm and pushing it back. Bend L knee, lift L heel and turn

hips and knee to R, weight on both legs equally. R hand to front of hip, elbow back, L arm down.
2-4 Deepen contraction. Fold L arm.

5-8 Stretch L leg, equal weight on both legs. Stretch L arm up diagonally with L leg. Accent.

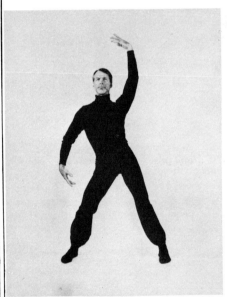 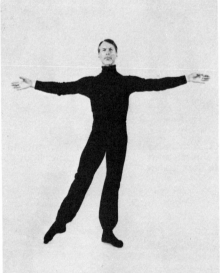 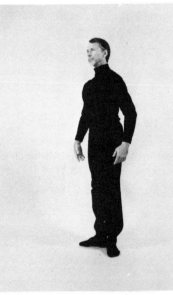

1 Turn body to front, standing in 2pp, flat feet, with R knee bent and weight equal. Contract L side and lift L hip diagonally up. Take arms shortest way to reverse S (high on L, low on R) with accent.
2-4 Deepen contraction on L side, keeping arms still.

5 Push weight onto L leg and turn out both legs. Stretch R leg to side, turned out. Arms to 2p.
6 Hold and enlarge position

7 Close R leg in 1p turned-out. Lower arms.
8 Hold and enlarge position.

Repeat from beginning to other side.

Repeat plié in 2p turned out.

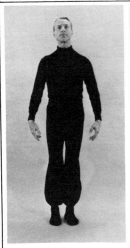 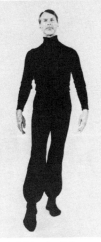 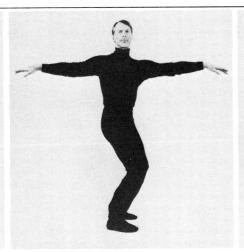 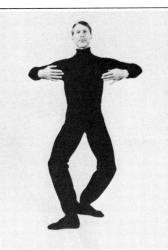

START in 1pp, arms down.

1-2 Tendu R leg forward parallel.

3-4 Turn feet to pt 7 (see space diagram, page 11) to small 2pp. Demi-plié, placing R foot on floor after pulling it closer to you. Arms to 2p, palms down.

5-6 Upper body still facing front, turn out R foot on heel to open 4p. Demi-plié, arms to 1p.

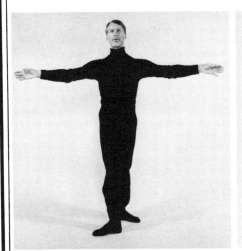 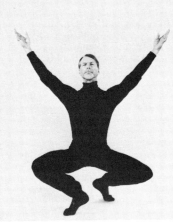 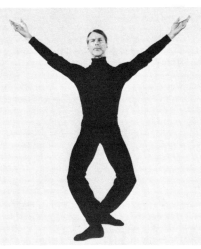

7-8 Straighten knees. Arms to 2p.

1-2 Grand plié in 4p, lifting head, chest and arms diagonally up. Palms slightly in.

3-4 Demi-plié in 4p, keeping head, chest and arms lifted.

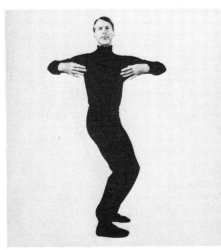 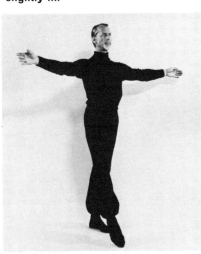 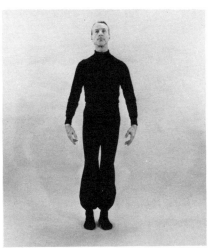

5 Turn R foot to parallel on heel. Arms to 1p.
6 Turn on heels to parallel forward, both heels on floor. Keep arms in 1p.

7 Push weight back to L leg. Stretch R leg forward parallel on floor. Arms to 2p.

8 Close R leg in 1pp. Lower arms. Repeat to front with L leg.

2. Pliés in 4th Position (page 2)

Do exercises with alternating legs en croix. To the side with right leg:

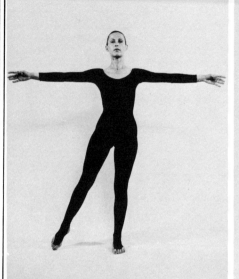

1-2 Tendu R leg to side parallel. Lift arms to 2p.

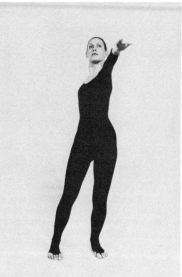

3-4 Place R foot on floor in a small 2pp, after pulling it a bit closer to you. Twist upper body to R, keeping head front. Palms down.

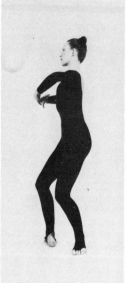

5-6 Turn out R foot on heel to open 4p. Demi-plié to pt.3. Arms to 1p. 7-8 Straighten knees. Arms to 2p.

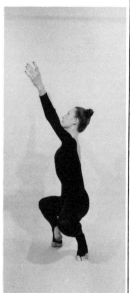

1-2 Grand plié in 4p, lifting chest, head and arms diagonally up. Palms slightly in.

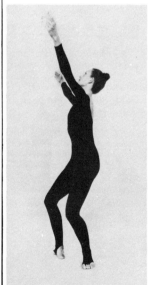

3-4 Demi-plié in 4p, keeping chest, head and arms lifted.

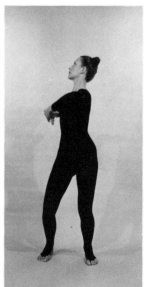

5-6 Turn R foot to parallel on heel. Arms to 1p.

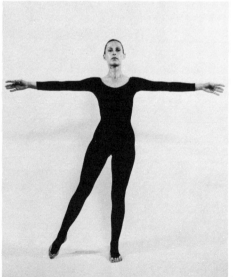

7 Facing front, push weight back to L leg, with R leg stretched parallel to the side, pointed foot on floor. Arms to 2p.

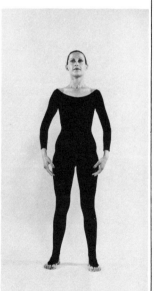

8 Close R leg in 1pp. Lower arms.

Do exercise to the side with left leg. Turn to pt 7 in grand plié.

Do exercise to the back. With right leg:

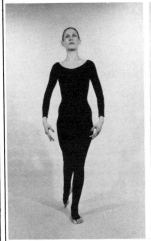 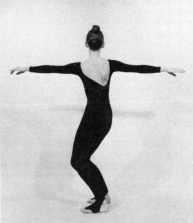 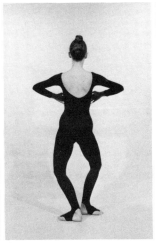 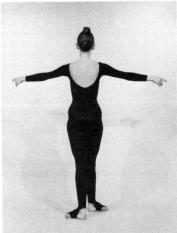

1-2 Tendu R leg back parallel.

3-4 Turn feet to pt 3 in small 2pp demi-plié. Twist upper body to R, arms lifted to 2p, palms down.

5-6 Turn out R foot on heel to open 4p. Demi-plié facing pt 5. Arms to 1p.

7-8 Straighten knees. Arms to 2p.

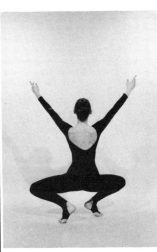 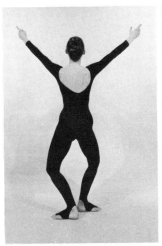 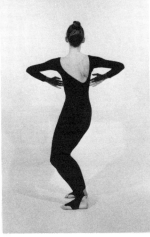 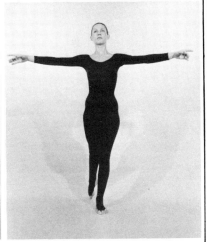

1-2 Grand plié in 4p, lifting chest, head and arms diagonally up. Palms slightly in.

3-4 Demi-plié in 4p, keeping chest, head and arms lifted.

5-6 Turn R foot to parallel on heel. Arms to 1p.

7 Facing front, push weight back to L leg with R leg stretched parallel to back, pointed foot on floor. Arms to 2p.

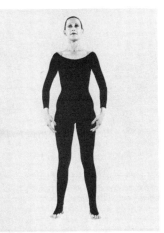

8 Close R leg in 1pp and lower arms.

Do exercises to the back with left leg.

A good exercise for the pointed foot, this sequence also helps you create a long, curved line with your body, as you lower your hip and raise your arm overhead. This line is used often in this style of dance. The exercise also gives you a sense of the demi-plié in another position.
— MM.

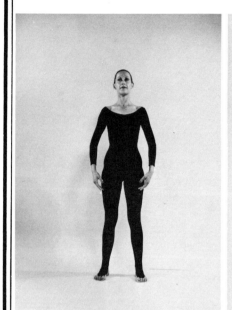

START in 1pp, arms down.

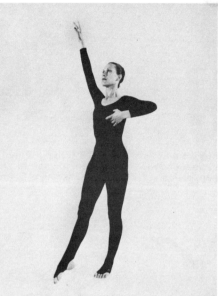

1-2 Tendu R leg forward parallel. Stretch R arm forward and up with palm starting back and finishing forward. L arm to 1p.

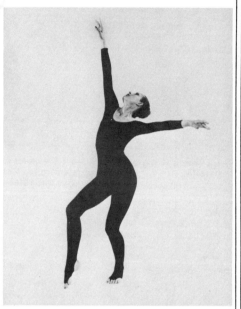

3-4 Bend both knees and contract L side, forcing hip out. Stretch through R side, lifting R shoulder. Look at R hand. Stretch L arm to 2p, twisting to L.

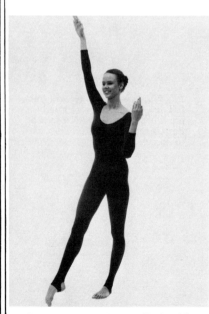

5 Straighten both knees. R shoulder to C with straight arm. Fold L arm.

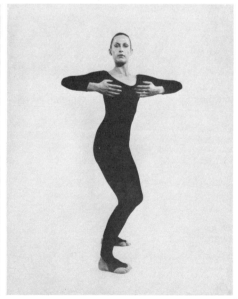

6 Fold R arm
AND Turn from waist down to pt 7 in small 2pp. Demi-plié. Bring arms to 1p.

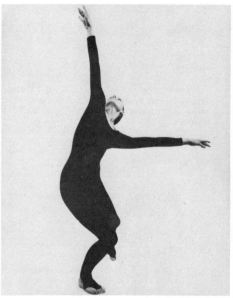

7-8 Place weight over R foot with L leg relaxed to side. Lean to L and stretch R arm up, leading with R shoulder. Finish with palm forward. Stretch through R side and lift R shoulder. L arm to L, palm down.

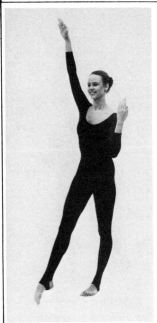

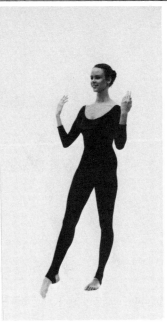

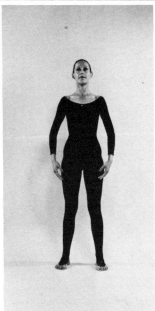

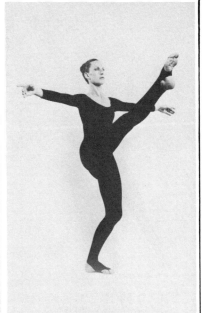

PART 1:
1-2 Turn body to front as you push weight over to L leg with R leg stretched forward on floor. Fold L arm.

3 Fold R arm.

4 Close R leg in 1pp and lower arms.

PART 2: With accent
5 Push R leg forward parallel with L leg in demi-plié. Arms to 2p.

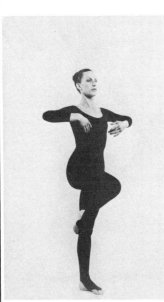

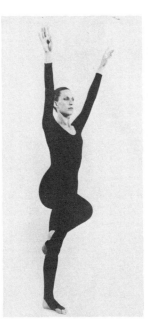

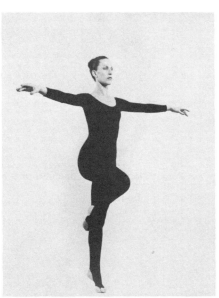

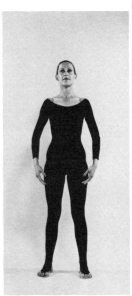

6 Stretch L leg and pull R leg in to passé parallel. Arms to lp.

AND Stretch arms up, palms forward.

7 Rise to half-toe on L leg. Arms to 2p, palms down.

8 Lower L heel as you place R leg in small 2pp. Lower arms.

3. Point Front #1 (page 3)

To the right with right leg:

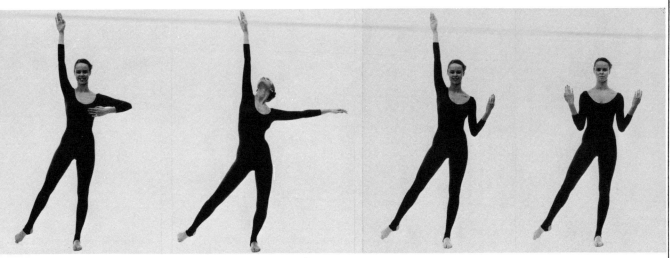

1-2 Tendu R leg to side parallel. Stretch R arm forward and up with palm starting back and finishing forward. L arm to 1p.
3-6 Continue exercise as to the front.

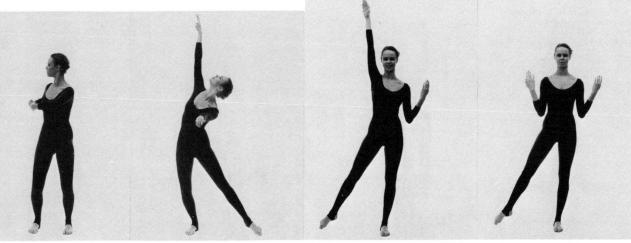

AND Place R leg in small 2pp demi-plié, and twist upper body to R. Arms to 1p.
7-8 Continue the sequence
1-4 as to the front.

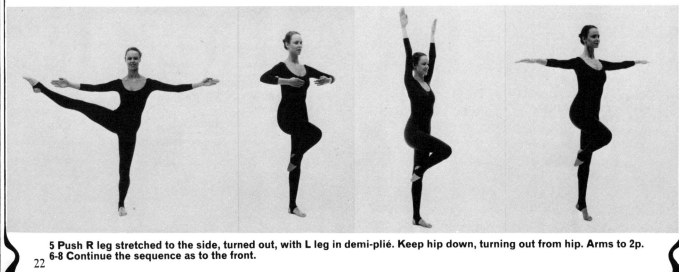

5 Push R leg stretched to the side, turned out, with L leg in demi-plié. Keep hip down, turning out from hip. Arms to 2p.
6-8 Continue the sequence as to the front.

To the back with right leg:

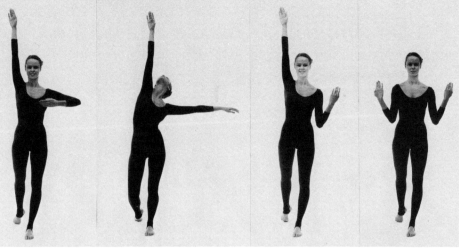

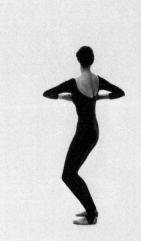

1-2 Tendu **R** leg back parallel. Stretch **R** arm forward and up with palm starting back and finishing forward. **L** arm to 1p.
3-6 Continue sequence as to the front.

AND Place **R** leg in a small 2pp demi-plié to pt 3. Twist upper body to the back. Arms to 1p.

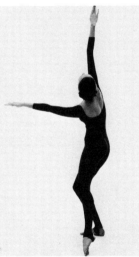

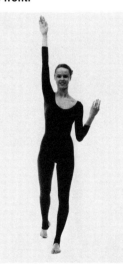

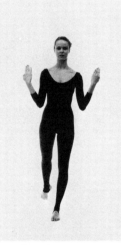

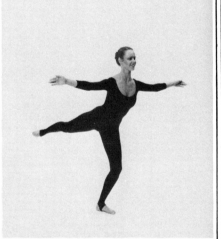

7-8 Stretch to the back as you did to the front.

1-2 Turn to front as you push weight to **L** leg. Stretch **R** leg back parallel on floor. Fold **L** arm.

3 Fold **R** arm.
4 Close **R** leg in 1pp. Lower arms.

5 Push **R** leg stretched to the back parallel with **L** leg in demi-plié. Arms to 2p.

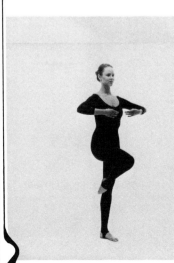

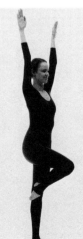

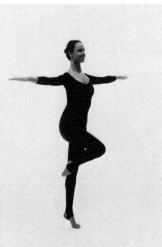

6-8 Continue the sequence as to the front, returning to 1pp, arms down.

This coordination exercise was developed for the training of the mind. It also develops the long leg line, the long body line while standing on one leg and—even more important—it develops the pointed foot, with a nice elongated arch.—MM.

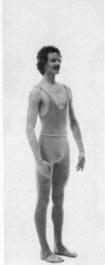 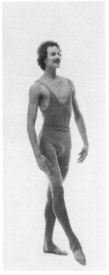 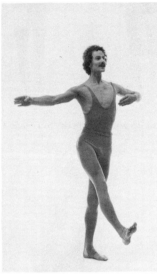 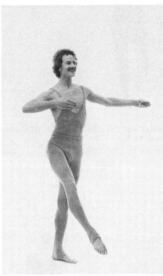 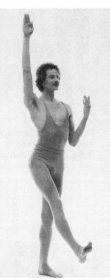

START in 1pp with arms down.

1-2 Tendu R leg parallel and close. **3-8** Repeat 3 times.

1 Push R leg stretched forward parallel, slightly off floor with flexed foot. L arm to 1p. R arm to 2p.

2 Point R foot. L arm to 2p. R arm to 1p.

3 Flex R foot. Fold L arm. Stretch R up with palm forward.

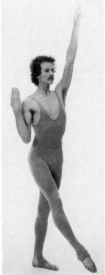 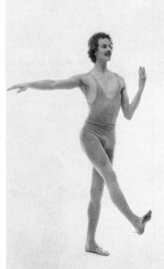 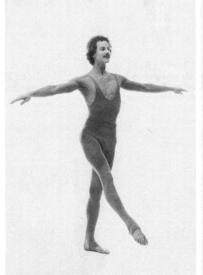 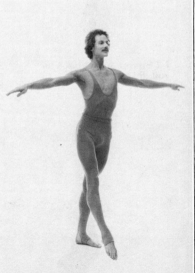

4 Point R foot. Stretch L arm up, palm forward. Fold R arm.

5 Flex R foot. Fold L arm. Take R arm to 2p, palm down.

6 Point R foot. L arm to 2p, palm down.

7 Point R foot on floor in front parallel. **8** Return to **START**.

Do exercise with alternating legs en croix. To the side: working leg is parallel in tendu *and turned out in flex/point. With right leg:*

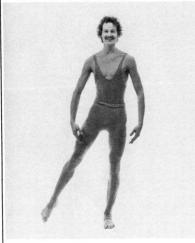

1-8 4 tendus and close to the side parallel.

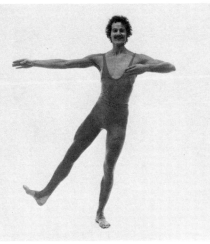

1 Push R leg stretched to the side, turned out, slightly off floor, foot flexed. L arm to 1p. R arm to 2p.

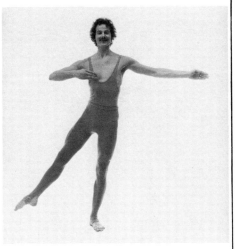

2-8 Continue the exercise—

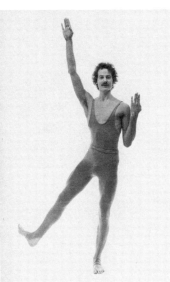

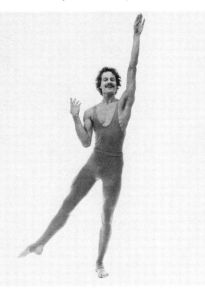

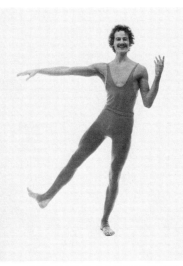

in the same way you did before to the front. Finish in starting position (first photo, page 24).

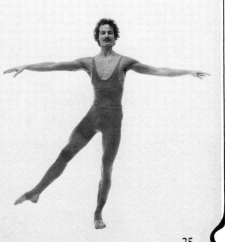

To the back, the working leg is parallel all the time. With the right leg:

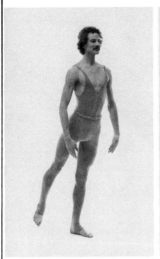

1-8 4 tendus and close to the back parallel.

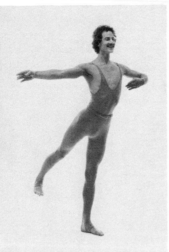

1 Push R leg, stretched to back parallel, slightly off floor, flexed foot. L arm to 1p. R arm to 2p.

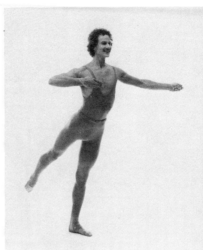

2-8 Continue the exercise—

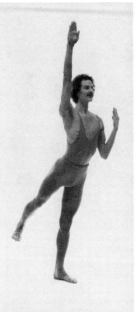

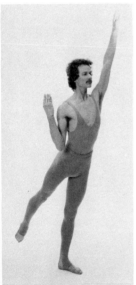

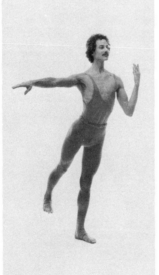

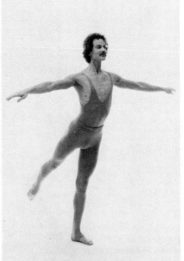

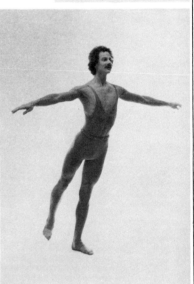

in the same way that you did to the front.

VARIATION: *Demi-plié on your standing leg on count 1. Straighten on count 2. Continue demi-plié and straighten on alternate counts, including count 6. Count 7 and 8 remain as before.*

On facing page: Elisabeth Frich

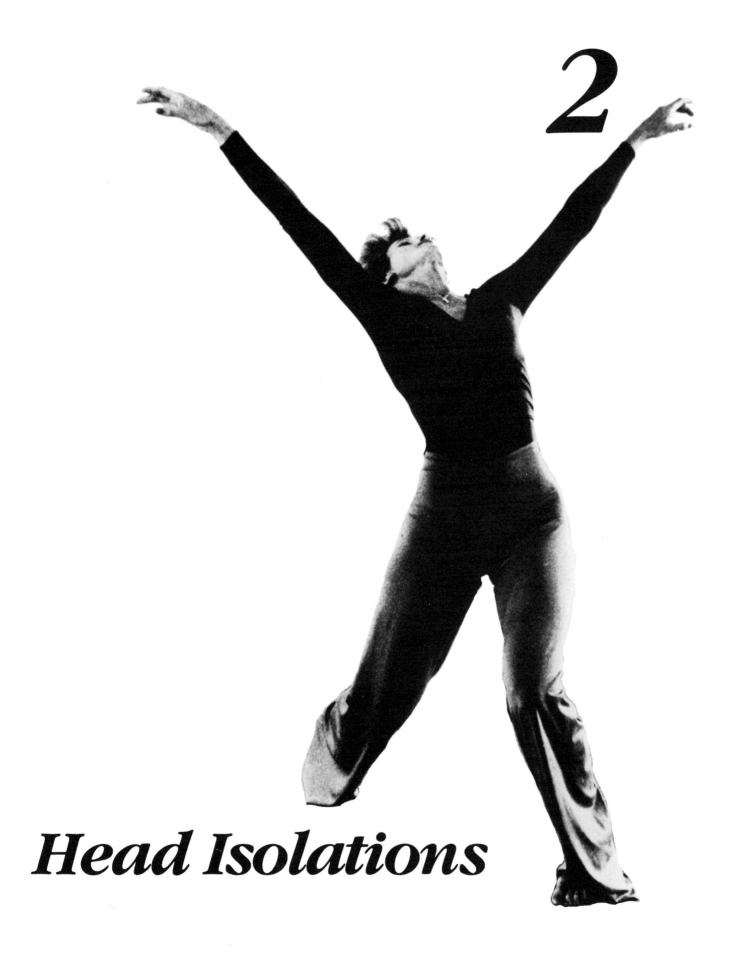

Head Isolations

2

The quick headroll is an excellent exercise for developing balance and control over your center. The stretch to the side is useful, too, with your arms going in counter-directions, one stretching up and away from the body, the other reaching down to the floor. At the same time, the exercise forces you to turn out while in a deep plié, which is fine for opening second position. Remember: At the moment you stretch to the side, press your knees well back and your pelvis well forward.—MM.

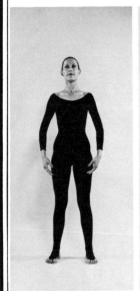 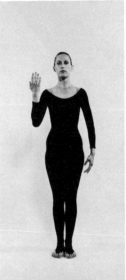 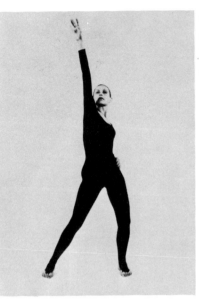 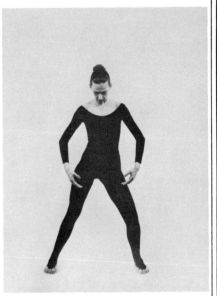

START in 1pp, arms down.

1-2 Fold R arm.

3. Stretch R arm up, palm forward, lifting R shoulder. Place L hand on L hip, elbow back. Twist to L slightly. Place straight R leg to side, flat foot, and bend L.

4 Hold and enlarge position. 5-8 Contract softly on R side and lift R hip diagonally. Bring R arm down through 2p. Finish with arms round, head down.

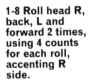 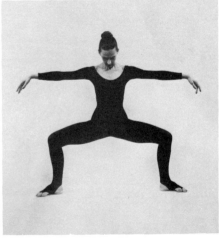 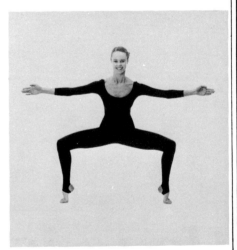

1-8 Roll head R, back, L and forward 2 times, using 4 counts for each roll, accenting R side.

AND Turn out and sit in grand plié 2p turned out. Drop head forward. Arms to 2p, hands relaxed.

1-8 Repeat headroll 4 times consecutively, using 2 counts for each roll, accenting R side.

1 Lift heels in grand plié, palms forward, head center. 2-4 Hold and enlarge position. 5 Lower heels and relax hands. 6-8 Deepen plié.

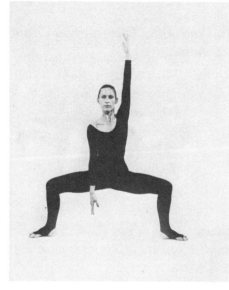

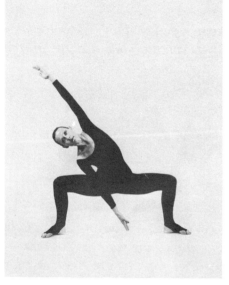

1 Stretch R arm down and L arm straight up, palms in.

2-8 Stretch upper body to the R in this position, pushing on the L side and keeping upper body aligned.

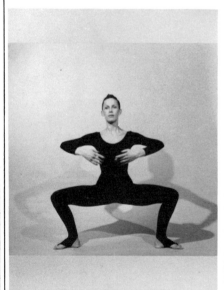

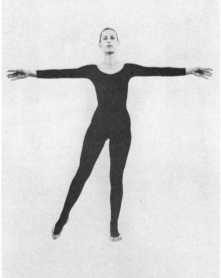

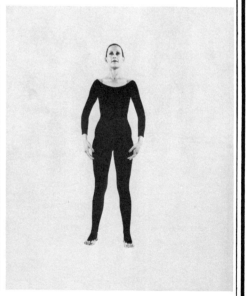

1-4 Upper body to C, arms to 1p.

5 Turn legs parallel as you push weight over to straight L leg, R leg stretched to side. Arms to 2p with force.
6 Hold and enlarge position.

7-8 Close R leg in 1pp. Lower arms.

Repeat from the beginning to the other side.

This exercise is designed to help coordinate head and arms. There are four distinct positions in it that you can use when making up combinations:

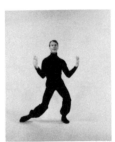 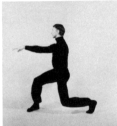 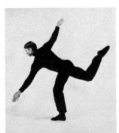 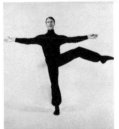

These major dance positions are particularly characteristic of jazz dance. This exercise is also effective for improving your leg positions—parallel and turned out. It also helps you with contractions, so important in this dance form.—MM.

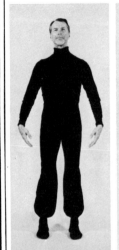 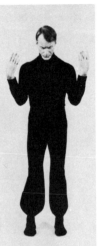 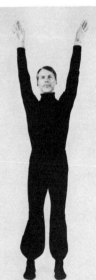 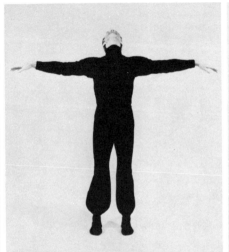 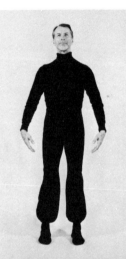

PART 1:
START in 1pp. arms down.

1 Drop head forward and fold arms.

2 Head to C. Arms up, palms forward (left).
3 Head back. Arms to 2p, palms down (above).

4 Head to C. Lower arms.
5-8 Repeat 1-4.

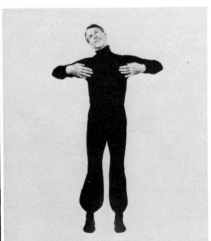 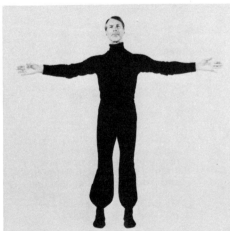 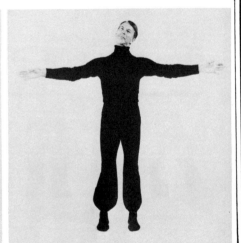

1 Tilt head to R, keeping face front, shoulders down. Arms to 1p.

2 Head to C. Arms to 2p.

3 Tilt head to L, face front.

30

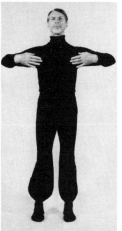

4 Head to C. Arms to 1p.

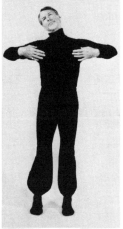

5 Tilt head to R.

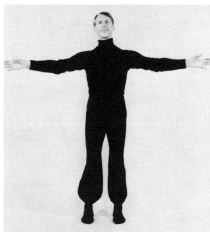

6 Head to C. Arms to 2p.

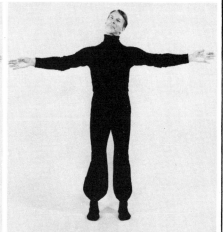

7 Tilt head to L.

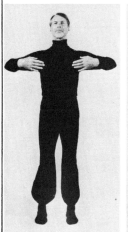

AND Head to C. Arms to 1p.

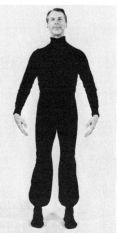

8 Lower arms.

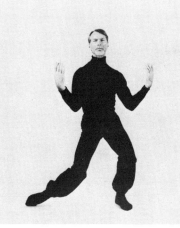

PART 2:
1 Place R leg relaxed to side. Fold arms. Lift elbows to 1p and start to shift weight to R leg.

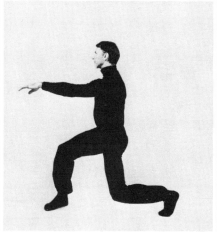

2 Turn to pt 3 in 4p turned in. Arms to 3p, middle. Accent.

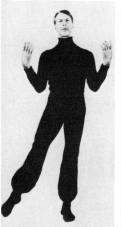

3 Face front, pushing weight to L leg. Stretch R leg parallel to side. Fold arms.

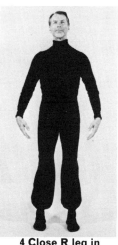

4 Close R leg in 1pp and lower arms.

5-8 Repeat last 4 counts (1-4) to L.

1-2 Repeat counts 1 and 2 (above) to R.

3 Place weight on R leg. Lift leg to parallel back attitude, facing pt 3. Twist upper body slightly to R. Stretch R arm up and L down on a diagonal line parallel to lower leg. Keep L hip down. Turn palms to back wall and look at L hand.

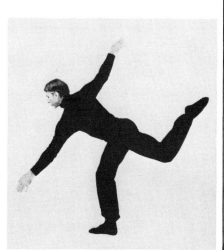

4-8 Hold and enlarge position.

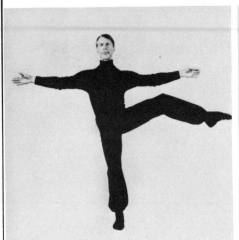

1 Turn body to front on **R** leg and turn out **L** leg to side in attitude. Arms to 2p.
2-8 Hold and enlarge position.

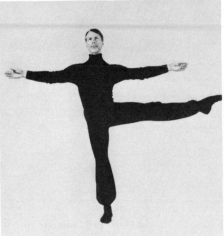

1-4 Straighten both knees.

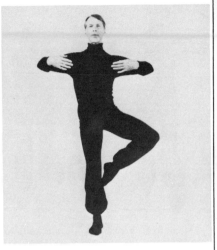

5 Pull in **L** leg to passé turned out. Arms to 1p.

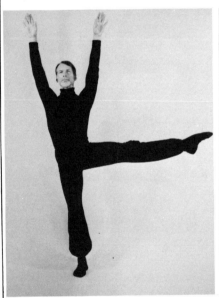

6 Stretch **L** leg to side, turned out. Arms up with palms forward.

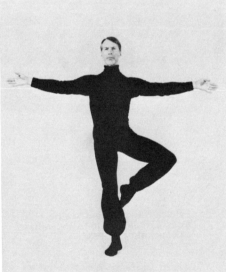

AND **Pull** in **L** leg to passé, turned out. Arms to 2p.

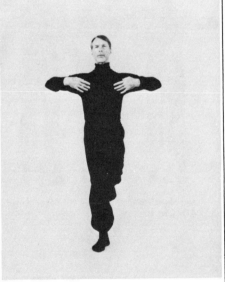

7 Turn **L** leg to passé parallel. Arms to 1p.
8 Close **L** leg in 1pp and lower arms, returning to starting position.

Repeat from the beginning to the other side.

6. Head Forward and Back/Right and Left (Tilt) (page 4)

Variation of PART *2.*

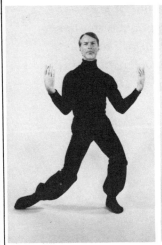

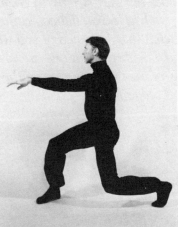

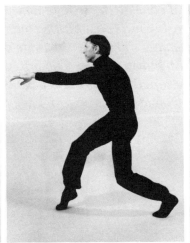

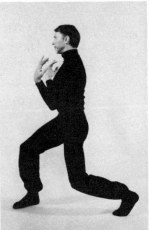

1 R leg to side relaxed. Fold arms, lift elbows to 1p. Start to shift weight to R leg.

2 Turn to pt 3 in 4p, turned in. Arms to 3p, middle. Accent.

3 Contract forward with accent. Lift both heels in 4p. 4 Hold and enlarge position.

5-6 Release and lower R heel. Fold arms.

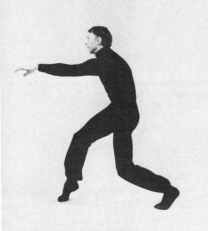

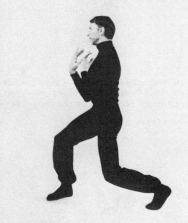

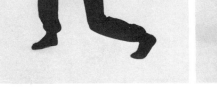

7-8 ⎫ Contract—release—contract—using 2 counts for each movement.
1-4 ⎭

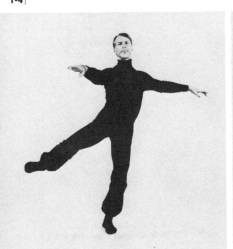

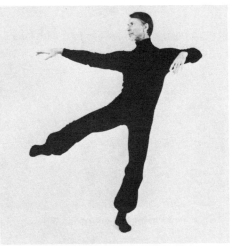

5 Turn body to front as you place weight on bent parallel L leg. Keep R leg in parallel side attitude. Arms 3p middle, R in front palms down. 6-8 Hold and enlarge position.

1 Lift L heel and turn head to R. R arm to 2p and L to 1p, with relaxed hands. 2-6 Hold and enlarge position.

7 Pull in R leg to passé parallel and straighten L leg. Fold arms.

8 Lower L heel and close R leg in 1pp. Lower arms.

33

7. Head Right and Left

Often in musical comedy the style of dance does not stay strictly in the realm of jazz—or classical—dance, but incorporates other forms, such as Indian dance, Siamese dance or other styles. These exercises will make you aware of what may be asked of you when you're called upon to do East Indian dance. The arm and kneeling positions are characteristic. This exercise also develops the control and flexibility of the neck muscles on the side, strengthens the thigh muscles and warms up hip, knee and ankle joints.—MM.

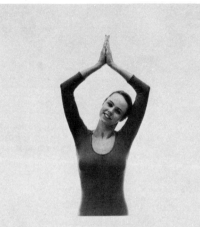

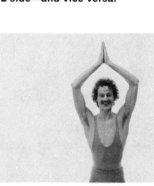

When you practice this exercise, do the head isolation from side to side in 1pp, arms overhead.

The best way to achieve a side-to-side isolation of the head is to tilt your head to the side (face front). Then push your chin sideways, parallel to the floor. When you push R, contract and shorten the muscles on the L side—and vice versa.

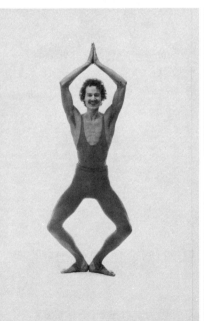

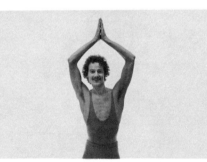

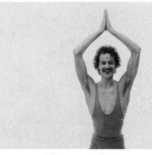

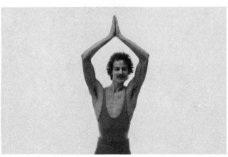

START in 1p turned out demi-plié, arms overhead, palms together.

1 Push head sideways to R with face front.

2 Push head to C.

3 Push head sideways to L.

4 Push head to C.
5-8 Repeat sequence 1-4.

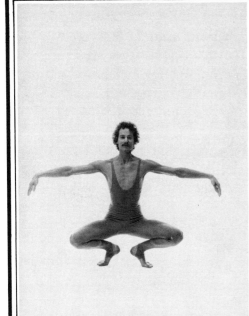

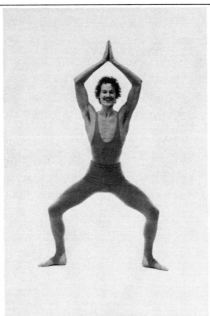

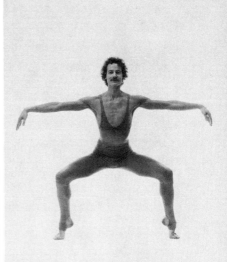

START
1 Grand plié, completely relaxed. Arms to 2p, relaxed hands.
2-4 Hold and enlarge position.

5 Open R leg to 2p, turned out grand plié. Arms overhead, palms together.
6-8 Hold and enlarge position.

1-2 Lift heels in grand plié, keeping at the same level. Arms to 2p, relaxed hands.
3-4 Lower heels.

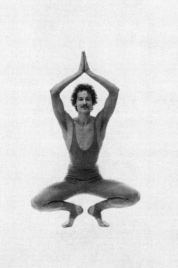

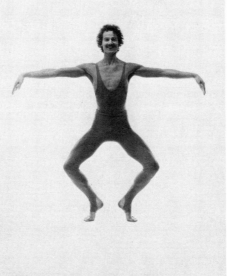

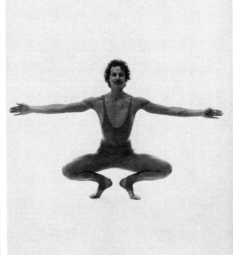

5 Return R leg to 1p, turned out grand plié, relaxed. Arms overhead, palms together.
6-8 Hold and enlarge position.

1 Demi-plié with heels lifted, arms to 2p, relaxed hands.
2 Hold and enlarge position.

3 Grand plié, relaxed, palms forward.
4 Hold and enlarge position.
5-8 Back to START.

Repeat from START *to the other side.*

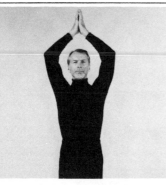

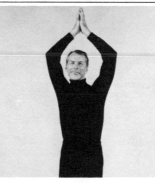

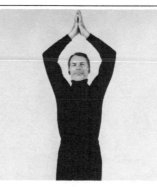

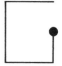

START in 1pp, arms overhead, framing face, palms together.

1-4 Push head forward in straight line, then R, then back—

and finally to C back.

You have just made a figure that looks like this:

5-8 Repeat from START to other side. On count 5 push head through C and forward.

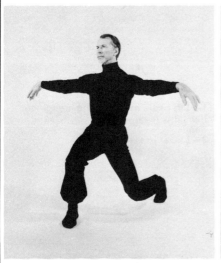

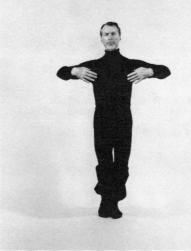

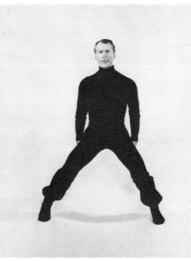

1 Step R leg forward into 4p turned in. Arms to 2p, relaxed hands. Push head forward.
2-8 Continue head isolation to R, then to L.

1 Push weight back and pull R leg to 1pp with lifted heel (no weight). Keep L leg bent, heel down. Arms to 1p.

AND Place R leg in wide 2pp with lifted heel, equal weight on each leg. Release through back and pelvis. Lower arms, passing slightly behind back.

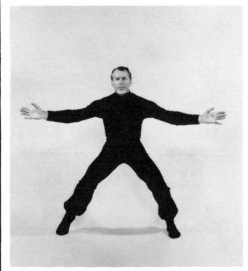

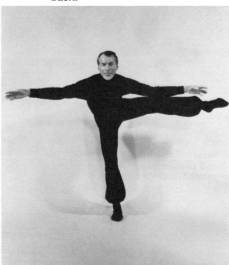

2 Contract forward and take arms to 2p. Accent.
3-4 Hold and enlarge position.

AND Softly return back and pelvis to C, arms to 1p.

5-8 Repeat release-
1-6 contraction 3 times with arms, using 4 counts for the first 2 and 2 counts for the 1 last.

7 Close R leg in 1pp with straight knees. Arms to 1p.

8 Arms to starting position.

VARIATION OF RELEASE-CONTRACTION: Place weight on bent R leg, with lifted heel. Lift L leg to parallel side attitude and softly lower R heel while you release and contract. Take upper body further forward. Repeat to other side.

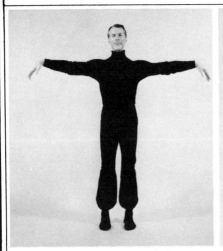

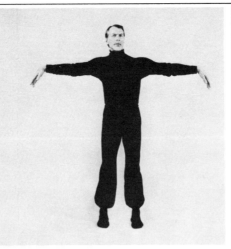

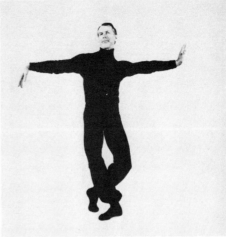

START in 1pp with arms in 2p, relaxed hands.

1-3 Push head forward and continue semi-circle to R, then back, parallel to floor, keeping face forward.

AND Place L foot, turned out, on half toe under R, slightly bent knees. Pull L shoulder blade in, lift L hand up, palm out.
4-6 Repeat semi-circle to L.

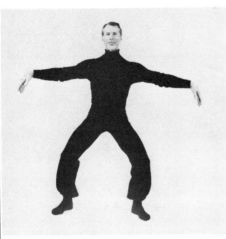

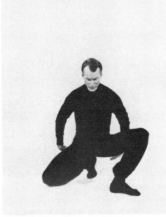

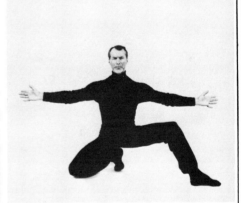

1 Step L leg to 2p, slightly turned out. Demi-plié. Bring L shoulder blade to C and L hand down.

2 Place R leg, turned out, back in 4p with lifted heel. Kneel on R knee, slightly turned out, equal weight on each leg, ball of R foot on floor. Take arms through 1p

and let them fall behind back, head forward.
3 Turn out L leg to side flat on floor with bent knees. Head to C, arms to 2p.

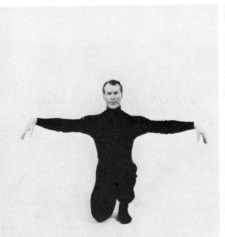

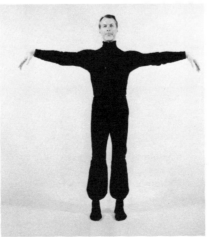

4 Pull in L leg and close both legs forward parallel. Relax hands.
5 Stand straight up on L leg.

6 Close R leg in 1pp and lower arms.

Repeat from the beginning to the other side.

On facing page: Matt Mattox

Shoulder Isolations

3

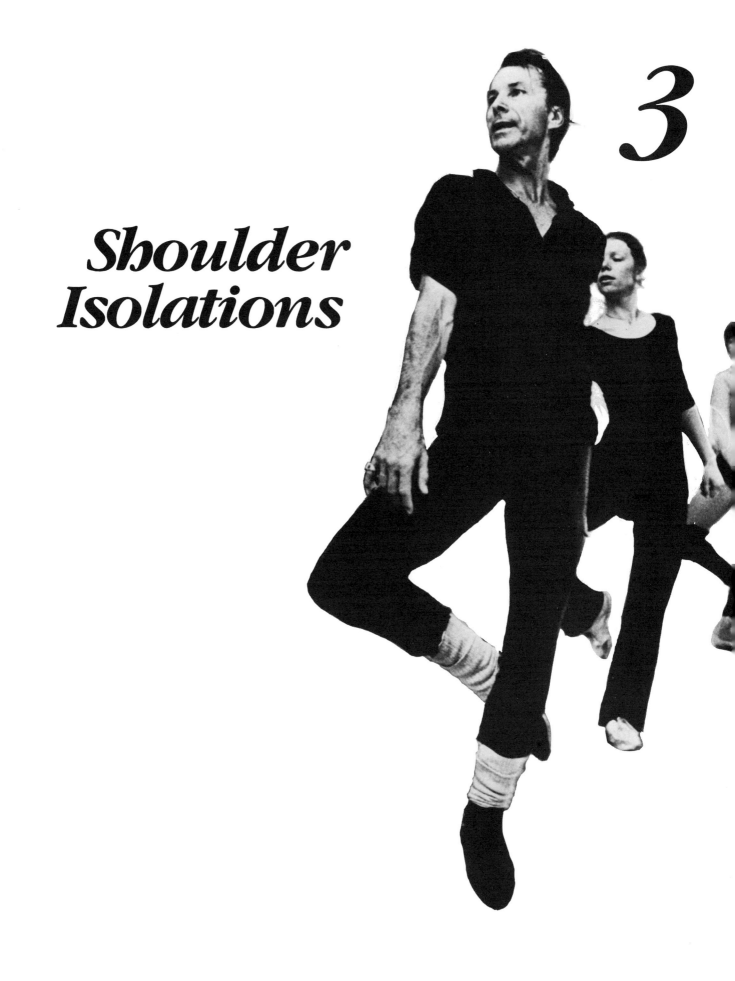

The primary reason for any warm-up is to prepare the body to work hard. With the following exercises, you'll learn not only to use your shoulders in any way you want at will, but you'll also warm up the joint of the shoulder and build the muscle structure into the condition it should have, in a well-exercised body.

Very often, the hands, arms and shoulders, muscularly, are used to make a rapid recovery from a prone position on the floor, or to make a quick fall to the floor from a standing position. These sequences will help you build up the strength in and around your shoulders so you can make those moves, besides teaching you how to isolate shoulder movements. These muscles are often forgotten when a warm-up is done, because so much of our concentration goes to the body, the legs and feet. Do these exercises daily.—MM.

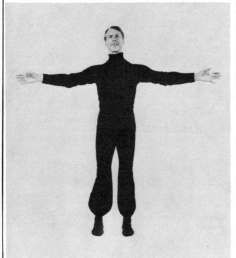

START in 1pp with arms in 2p.

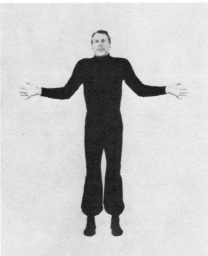

1 Lift both shoulders straight up.

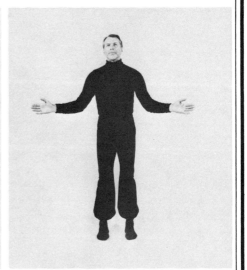

2 Push shoulders forward and down.
3 Lift both shoulders up—
4 and then to C.
5-8 Repeat from START.

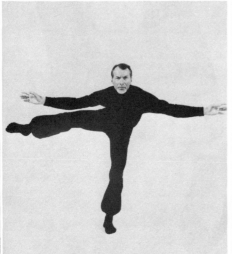

1-4 Repeat from START with forward contraction. Lift R leg to parallel side attitude on count 2, taking upper body further forward, L leg bent.
5-8 Repeat last 4 counts to other side.

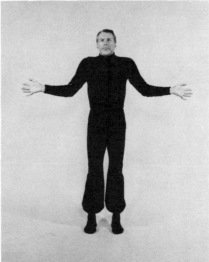

1 Lift both shoulders straight up.

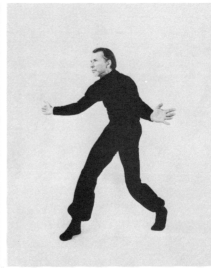

2 Push shoulders forward and down with forward contraction. Step R leg forward to 4p turned in.
3-4 Lift both shoulders. Return to 1p, bringing them to C.
5-8 Repeat last 4 counts to other side.

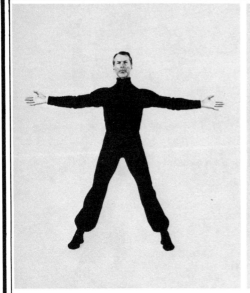

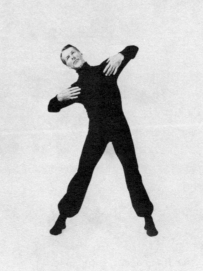

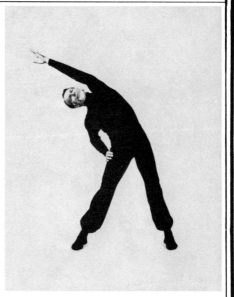

1 Place R leg in 2 pp with straight knees. Arms to 2p.

2 Arms to 1p.
AND Stretch upper body to R.

3 Place R hand on R thigh. Stretch L arm up along L side of head. Stretch through L side, looking in direction of hand.
AND 4 Reverse, return to START.

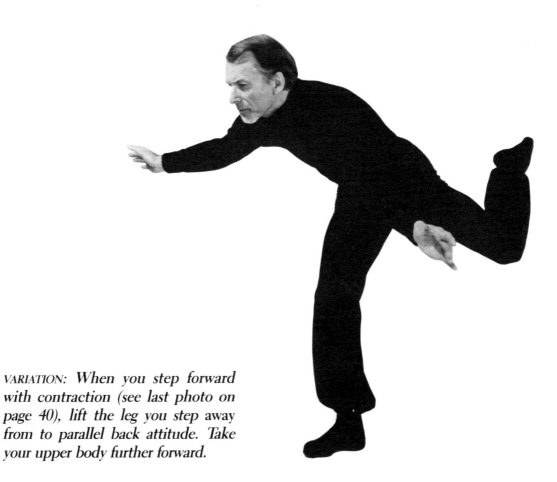

VARIATION: When you step forward with contraction (see last photo on page 40), lift the leg you step away from to parallel back attitude. Take your upper body further forward.

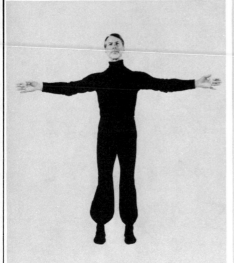

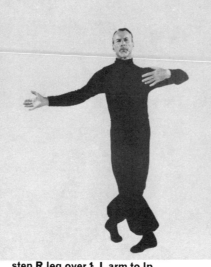

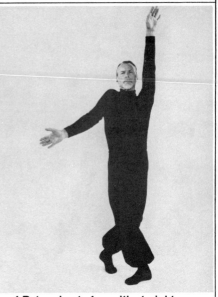

PART 1:
START in 1pp with arms in 2p.
1 Lift R shoulder straight up.
2 Push it forward and down as you

step R leg over †, L arm to lp.
3 Lift shoulder and stretch L arm up,
palm forward.

4 Return leg to 1pp with straight
knees. L arm to 2p.
5-8 Repeat from START to other side.

Repeat from the beginning, but step under the leg.

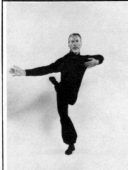

VARIATION OF PART 1

Lift leg you step away from to back attitude,
as you push shoulders forward and down.
Move forward and back to 1pp.
_____

Step R leg over L. Lift L leg to parallel back
attitude. Same with L leg (over R) to parallel
back attitude.

Step R leg under L.
Lift leg to turned out
forward attitude.
Same with L leg
(under R).

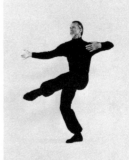

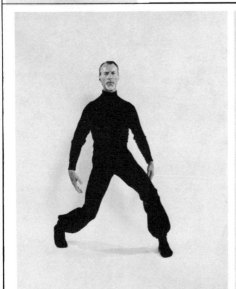

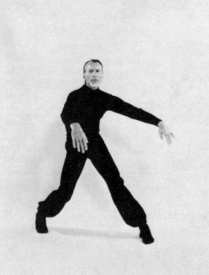

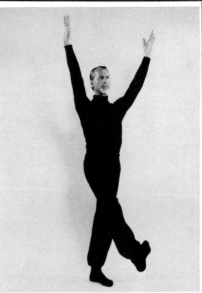

PART 2:
1 Place R leg in 4p turned in facing pt
8. Let arms fall.

2-6 While stretching L leg, do forward
contraction, stretch arms forward,
palms down.

7–8 Turn to front. Take R leg straight
through 1pp without putting weight on
it and bring it forward with flexed
foot. Palms in.

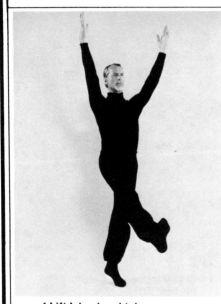

1 Lift L heel and take arms up, palms in.
2-6 Hold and enlarge position.
7 Fold arms, lower L heel.
8 Close R leg in 1pp. Lower arms.

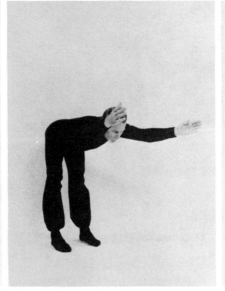

1 Stretch arms forward and up, palms in. Lift well up from waist.
2 Stretch body forward at 90° angle, straight back.

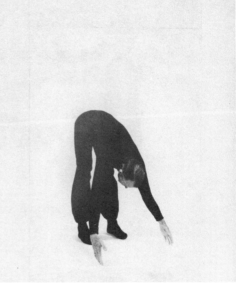

3 Stretch diagonally down at 45° angle.
4 Roll up, vertebra by vertebra to standing position.
5-8 Repeat last 4 counts.

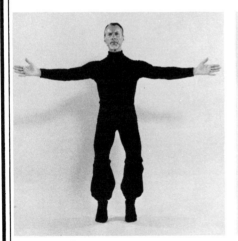

PART 3:
1 Demi-plié, arms in 2p, palms forward.
2 Lift heels, keeping pelvis still (above).
3 Straighten knees, turn palms down.
4 Lower heels and arms.
5-8 Repeat last 4 counts.

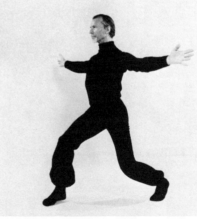

1-2 Place R leg in 4p, turned in to pt 2, arms in 2p.
AND Release softly (above), keeping arms still.

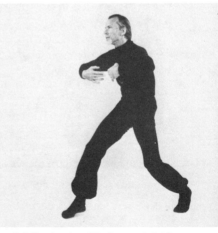

3-4 Contract softly forward, taking arms to 1p.
AND 5-8 Change direction to pt 8 without moving feet and repeat release/contract. Repeat last 4 counts to R/L.

Repeat from Part 1 to the other side.

12. One Shoulder Against the Other + Shimmy   clean, crisp movements

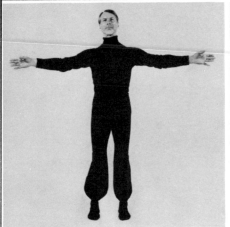

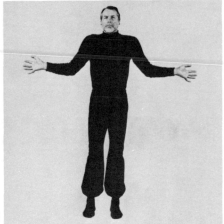

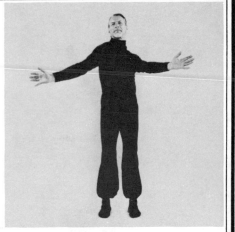

START in 1pp with arms in 2p.

1 Lift both shoulders straight up.

2 Push R shoulder forward and down. Move L shoulder back and down.
3 Lift shoulders up
4 and to C.
5-8 Repeat from START to other side.

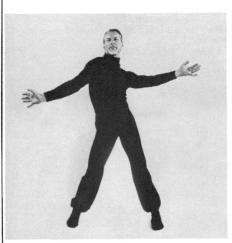

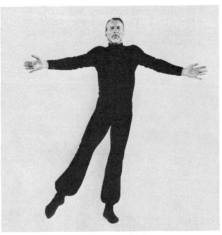

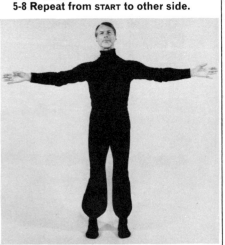

1 Lift both shoulders up (middle picture above).
2 Push R shoulder forward and down as before, but step to R on bent leg parallel, flat foot. Contract L side, lift L hip diagonally, chest front. Accent.

3 Lift up shoulders and push weight over to L leg. Point R foot to side parallel.

4 Close R leg in 1pp. Shoulders to C.
5-8 Repeat last 4 counts to other side.

1-6 Place R leg in 2pp demi-plié and shimmy with arms in 2p.

7-8 Close R leg in 1pp and lower arms.

1 Stretch both arms forward and up with palms in. Lift heels.

2 Hold and enlarge position.

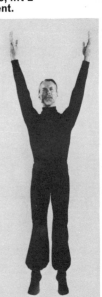

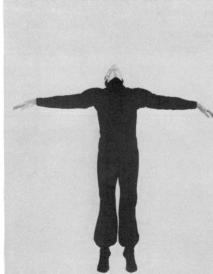

3 Bend back, taking arms to 2p, palms down.
4 Hold and enlarge position.

5 Upper body to C.

6 Hold and enlarge position.

7 Lower heels and arms.

8 Hold and enlarge position.

1-8 Repeat last 8 counts.

Repeat from beginning to other side.

Ribcage
Isolations

4

This exercise is designed to help you move your ribcage at will. A major coordination, it is also an essential movement in the "ripple." When you master this exercise, you'll have mastered the basic "ripple" movement. Arm movements here are strictly for coordination—and the training of the mind.—MM.

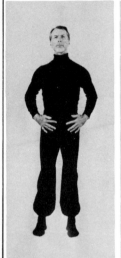 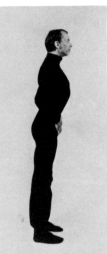 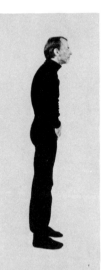 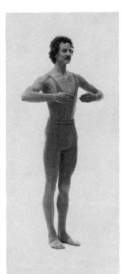 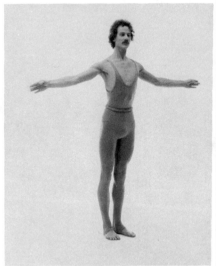

START in 1pp, hands on front of hips.

1-2 Push ribcage forward (above) and then back to C.

3-4 Push ribcage back (above) and then back to C.

5-8 Repeat 1-4. On 8 take arms to 1pp (above).

1 Push ribcage forward. Arms to 2p with flip hands.

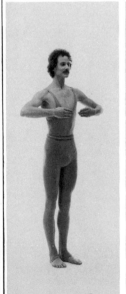 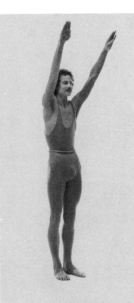 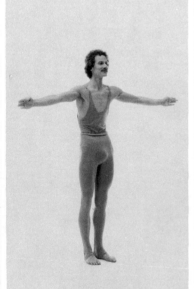 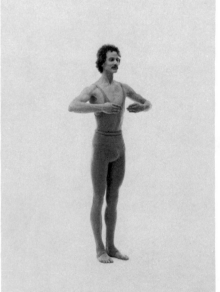

2 Push ribcage to C. Arms to 1p.

3 Push ribcage back. Stretch arms up, palms forward.

AND Arms to 2p.

4 Push ribcage to C. Arms to 1p. 5-8 Repeat last 8 counts.

Place hands on front of hips as you repeat from the beginning.

A coordination exercise, this sequence also helps you to isolate the ribcage, a common movement in many forms of jazz dance. It also incorporates the forward/backward action of the "ripple."—MM.

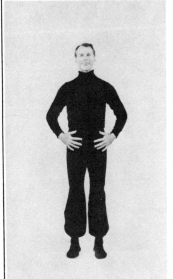

START in 1pp, hands on front of hips.

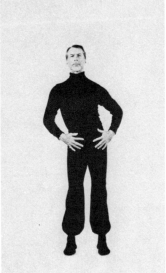

1-2 Push ribcage to R (above) and back to C.

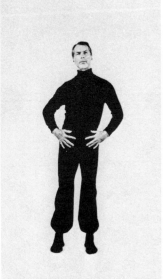

3-4 Push ribcage to L (above) and to back and C.
5-8 Repeat 1-4.

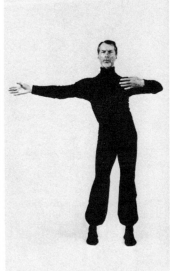

1 Push ribcage R. Bring R arm to 2p. Bring L arm to 1p.

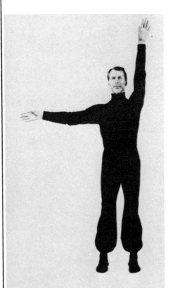

2 Push ribcage to C. Stretch L arm up, palm forward along side of head.

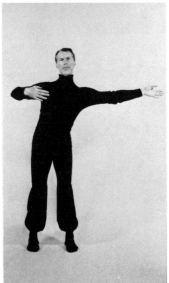

3 Push ribcage L. Bring L arm to 2p, R arm to 1p.

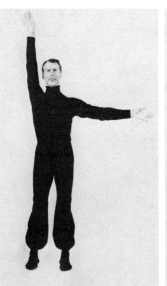

4 Push ribcage to C. Stretch R arm up, palm forward along side of head.
5-8 Repeat last 4 counts.

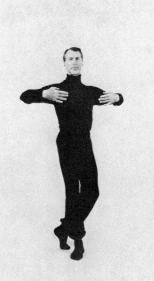

1 Place L foot under R on half-toe, L leg bent, both legs slightly turned out. Turn body to pt 8. Arms to 1p.

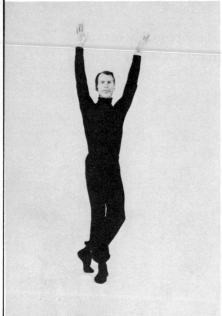

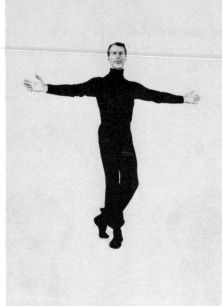

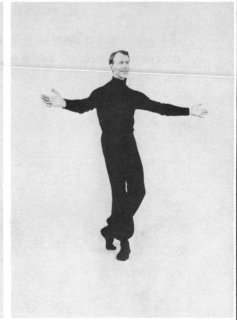

2 Hold and enlarge position.
3 (above) Stretch both arms up, palms forward.
4 Hold and enlarge position.

5-8 Arms to 2p, palms forward.

1 Contract hip forward.

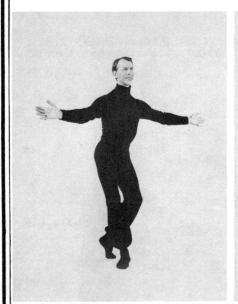

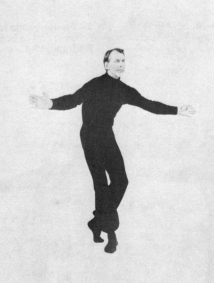

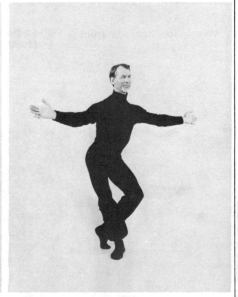

2 Release hip back.

3-4 Contract your ribcage back as you contract hip forward.

5-6 Release ribcage forward as you release hip back.
7 Close L leg in 1pp to pt 1.
8 Hold and enlarge position.

Note: In 3-6 you create 2 soft ripples while you deepen the demi-plié, keeping arms still.

Repeat from the beginning to the other side.

This exercise is similar to the last, but it is especially effective for the training of the mind—and the coordinating of body and arm movements.—MM.

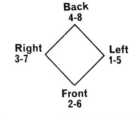

Back
4-8

Right
3-7

Left
1-5

Front
2-6

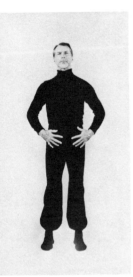 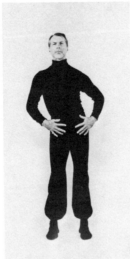 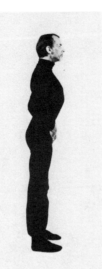 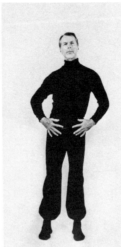 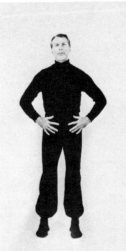

START in 1pp, hands on front of hips.

1-16 Push ribcage
–R–   –front–   –L–   –back–
and then L, front, R and back 2 times in the pattern of a diamond (see above), using one count for each movement.

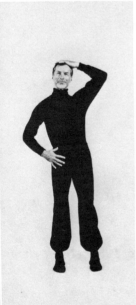 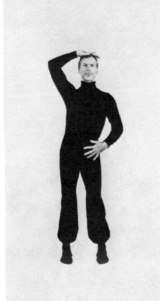 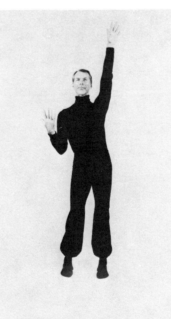 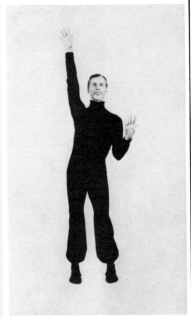

1 Place L hand on head with palm down. Push ribcage R.
2-4 Push ribcage front, left and back.

5 Place L hand on front of L hip, R hand on head, palm down. Push ribcage L.
6-8 Push ribcage front, R and back.

1-8 Repeat last 8 counts.
1 Fold R arm, stretch L arm up shortest way, palm forward. Push ribcage R.
2-4 Push ribcage forward, L and back.

Stretch R arm up, palm forward. Fold L arm. Push ribcage L.
5-8 Push ribcage front, R, back.

Repeat from the beginning to the other side.

On facing page: Elisabeth Frich

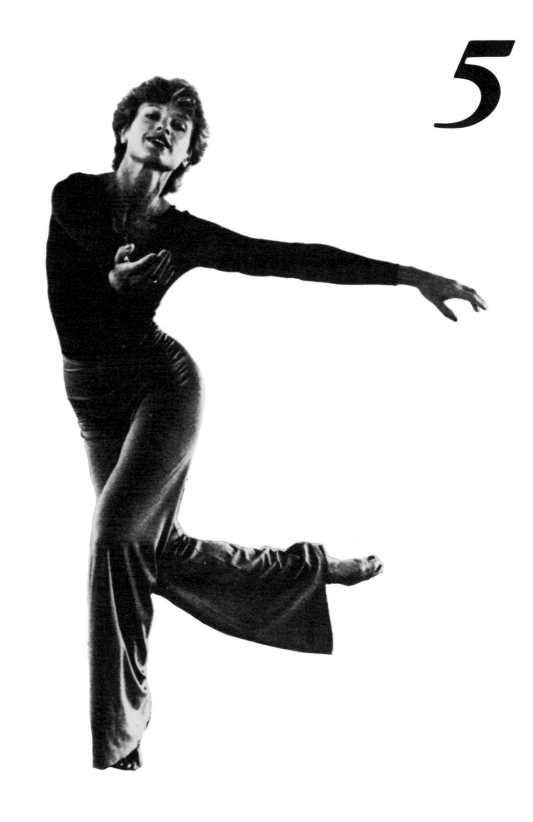

Pelvis Isolations

Pelvis Isolations

The following exercises aid in creating coordination of head, body and arms, but more important, they give a working knowledge necessary for many pelvic movements in jazz dance. The "bump and grind," as it was called in burlesque in the early days, was used to create a sensual reaction from the men who watched it done by the female artists of striptease. This connotation still exists today when we do the pelvic roll: the right/front/left/back and reverse movements of the pelvis, with head and arms working as well, and the quick push of the pelvis into place, resting there for the second count.

I designed this exercise for jazz dancers, because women particularly are called upon often to impersonate striptease artists, and there is no better place to learn how to do it than in a dance class.

Again, all these isolations are meant to make dancers work their brains and coordinate their bodies, so that their capacity for adaptability—to any style of dance—is possible. And, never let it be forgotten that we are warming up the entire anatomy as well, preparing the body for its ultimate task and that is to dance.—MM.

16. Hip Rotation   long, smooth movements

In this exercise, the pelvis is pushed softly in a horizontal circle and a figure 8—both halves of which go to the side, not forward and back.—MM.

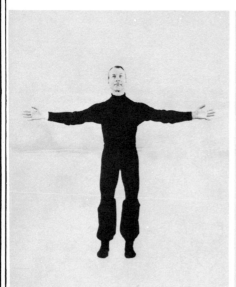 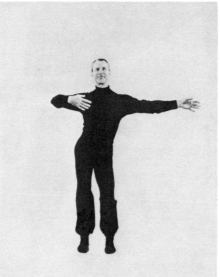 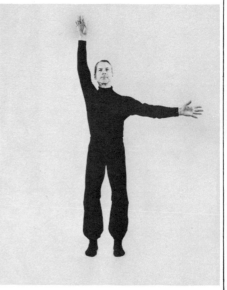

PART 1:
START in 1pp demi-plié with arms in 2p.

1-2 Push hip to R and take R arm to 1p.
AND Turn R palm forward.

3-4 Push hip forward and stretch R arm up along R side of head.

16. Hip Rotation (page 2)

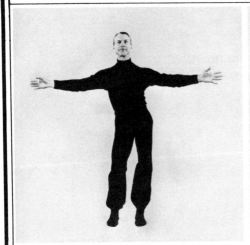

5-6 Push hip L. Take R arm to 2p.

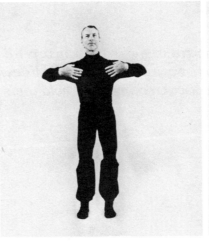

7 Push hip back
AND Arms to 1p.
8 Arms to 2p, with flip hands.

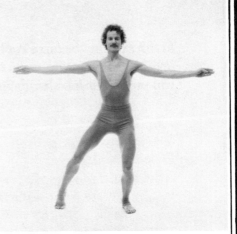

1-8 Repeat from START with R leg bent parallel to the side on the ball of the foot.
1-16 Repeat from START to L.

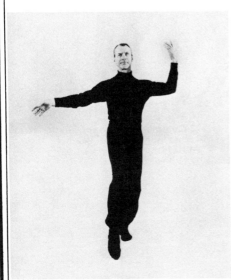

PART 2:
AND Place R leg forward, relaxed.
1-2 Start ½ horizontal figure 8: pushing hip diagonally forward and R.

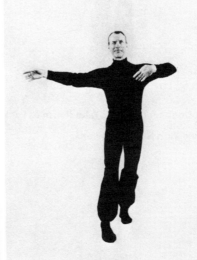

3-4 Close R leg in 1pp as you finish figure 8 diagonally R back. Make 1 inward circle with L lower arm on last 4 counts.

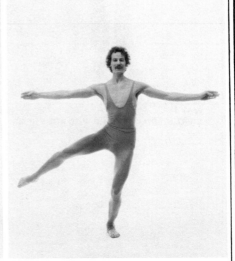

Repeat from START to other side.
VARIATION (above): Lift leg to parallel side attitude during second half of PART 1.

PART 1

Back 7-8

Right 1-2   Center   Left 5-6

Front 3-4

PART 2

Back

Right 1-4   Left 5-8

Front

In this exercise the hip is contracted sharply in the pattern of a diamond: R/F/L/Back. It is the same rotation as in Part 1 of Exercise 16, except that you push your hip sharply in place on count 1 and hold count 2.

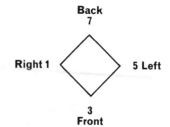

Back 7

Right 1   5 Left

3 Front

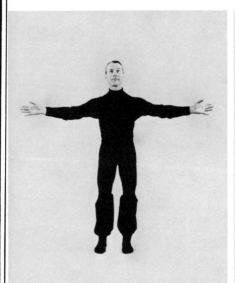

PART 1:
START in 1pp demi-plié with arms in 2p.

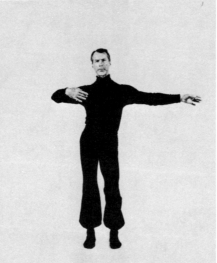

1 Contract hip to R. Take R arm to 1p.
2 Hold.
AND Turn R palm forward.

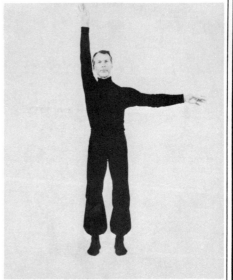

3 Contract hip forward. Stretch R arm along R side of head.
4 Hold.

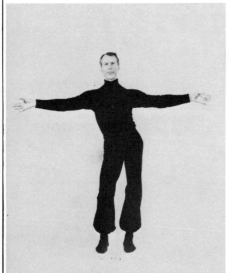

5 Contract hip L and take R arm to 2p.
6 Hold.

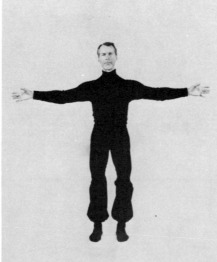

7 Release hip back.
AND Arms to 1p.
8 Arms to 2p with flip hands.

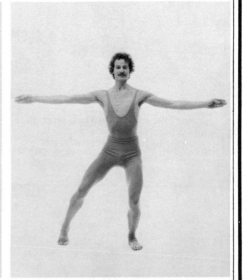

1-8 Repeat from START with R leg bent parallel to side.
AND Close R leg in 1pp demi-plié.
1-16 Repeat from START to L.

On to part 2—

54

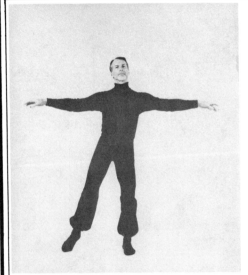

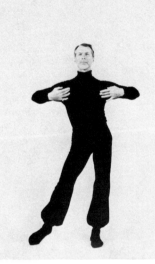

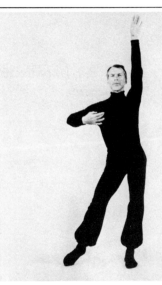

PART 2:
AND Close L leg in 1pp, demi-plié, and place **R** leg bent parallel to side with lifted heel. Palms down.

1 AND Contract hip to **L**. Release it back to starting position. Rotate **R** lower arm in one outward circle. **L** arm to 1p.

2 AND Repeat contract/release of hip. Turn **L** palm forward. Stretch **L** arm up along **L** side of head. Do one outward circle with lower arm.

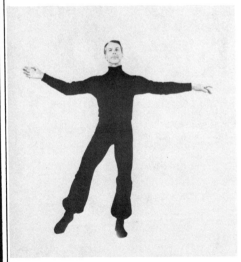

AND Close R leg in 1pp, demi-plié. Finish **R** arm in 2p as you release hip.

5-8 Repeat PART 2 to other side.

1-8 Repeat from start of **PART 2**.

3 AND 4 Repeat contract/release/contract, repeating arm action twice with **R** arm and taking **L** arm to 2p, palm down.

Variations (below)

(Left): Lift leg to parallel side attitude.

(Center): Or keep it relaxed to side and add head movement in Part 2. As you contract/release hip to **L** 4 times, drop head forward in 2 counts and take it back to **C** in 2 counts.

(Right): As you contract/release hip to the **R** 4 times, drop head back in 2 counts and take it back to **C** in 2 counts. Continue the circling of the arm.

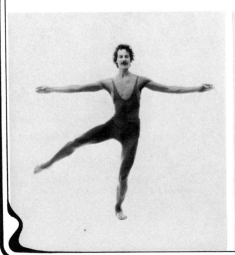

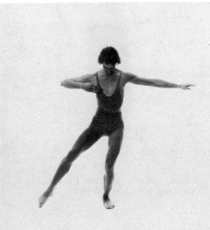

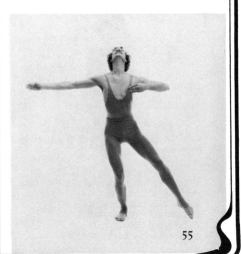

In this exercise the hip is contracted sharply in the pattern of a diamond (PART 1) and a cross (PART 2).

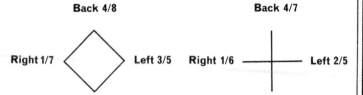

Back 4/8   Back 4/7

Right 1/7   Left 3/5   Right 1/6   Left 2/5

Front 2/6   Front 3/8

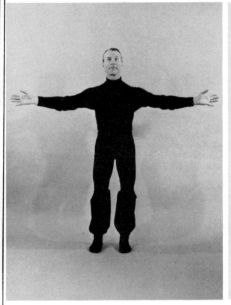

PART 1:
START in 1pp, demi-plié, arms in 2p.

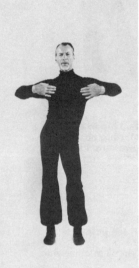

**1 Contract hip to R.
Close arms in 1p.**

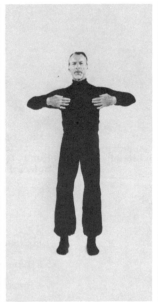

2 Contract hip forward.

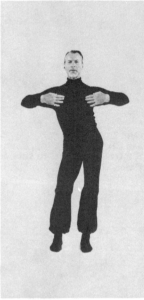

3 Contract hip to L.

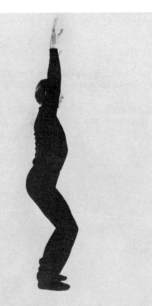

**4 Release hip back and stretch arms up, palms forward.
5 Contract hip L, arms up.
6 Contract hip forward.
7 Contract hip R.
8 Release hip back, arms 2p.**

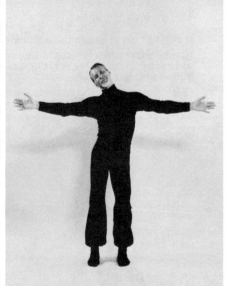

PART 2:
1 Contract hip to R and tilt head to R, keeping shoulders down.

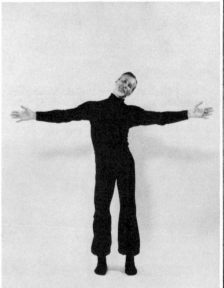

2 Contract hip to L. Tilt head L without stopping in C.

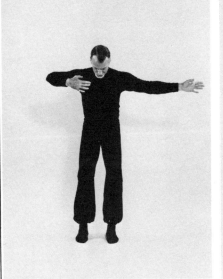

3 Contract hip forward and let head drop forward. **R arm 1p.**

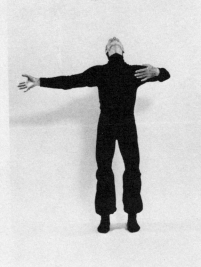

4 Release hip back and lift head back. **R arm 2p. L arm 1p.**

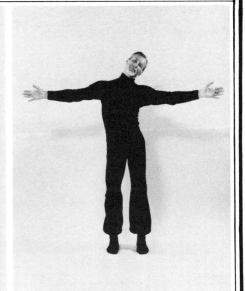

5 Contract hip L. Tilt head L. **L arm 2p.**

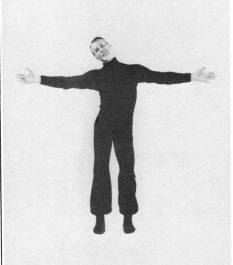

6 Contract hip **R.** Tilt head **R** without stopping in **C.**

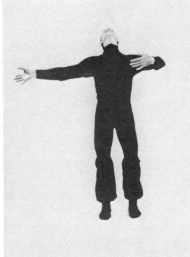

7 Release hip back; lift head back. **L arm to 1p.**

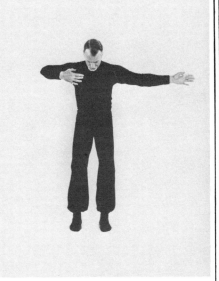

8 Contract hip forward. Let head drop forward. **R arm 1p. L arm 2p.**

Move head to Center and move Left arm to 1p to start repeating sequence from the beginning to the other side.

VARIATION: *Do sequence in ¾ rhythm 1 AND 2*

3

4 AND 5

6

On facing page: Matt Mattox and Elisabeth Frich

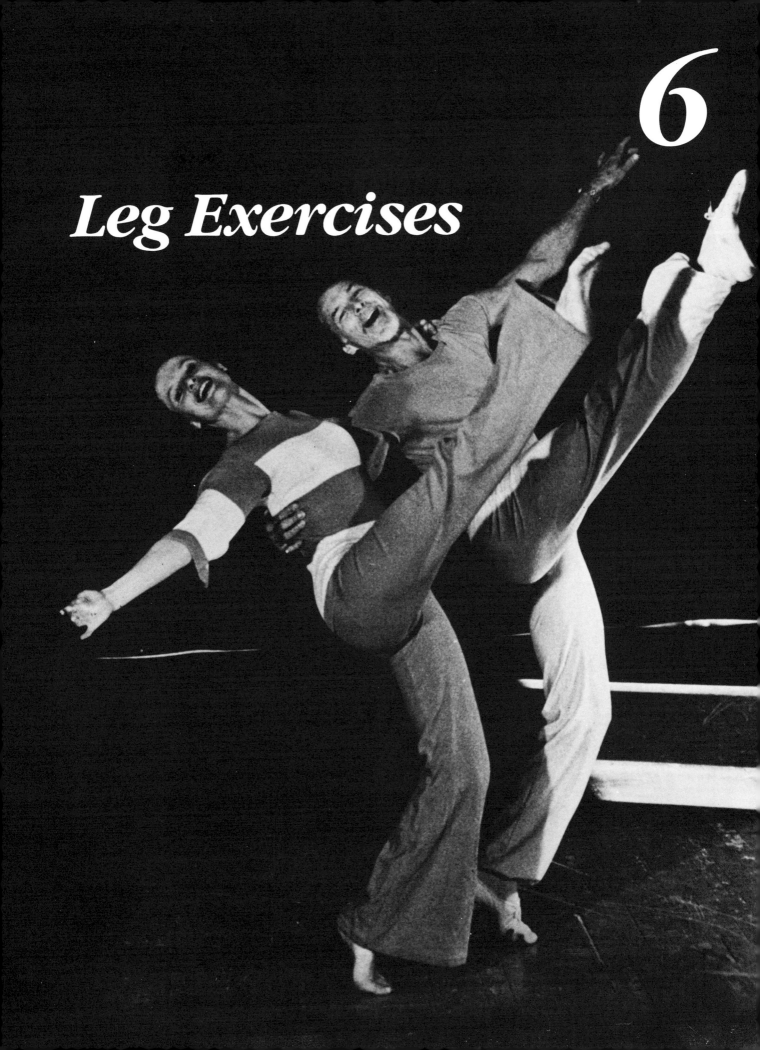

Leg Exercises

6

19. Point Flex, Point and Down

When you force your heel forward in this exercise, and bring your toes back—with your leg in a contraction—you will be forced to get your knee in the right position to create a long leg line. Besides this, the exercise makes you aware of the difference between the pointed foot and the flexed foot, and it helps you to balance on one leg. Moving your head at the moment of balance calls for added concentration in order to keep your center of gravity.—MM.

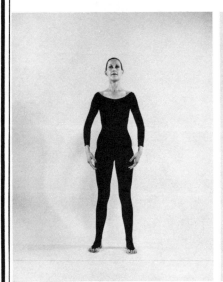

START in 1pp, arms down.

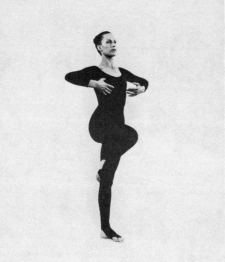

1 Lift **R** leg sharply to passé parallel.
Arms 1p.
2-4 Hold and enlarge position.

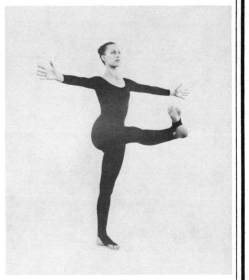

5-8 Softly extend **R** leg forward, flexed foot. Arms 2p.

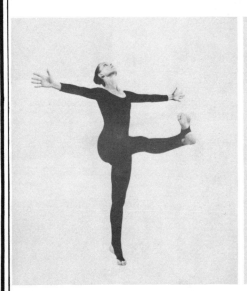

1-4 Rise to half-toe **L** leg, lift head back.

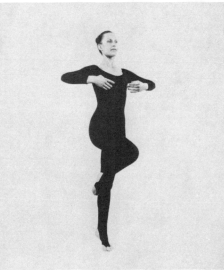

5-6 Pull in **R** leg to passé parallel on balance. Head C. Arms 1p.

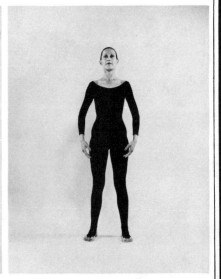

7-8 Lower arms and **L** heel as you place **R** leg in 1pp.
Do exercise with alternating legs en croix.

Do the exercise with alternating legs en croix:

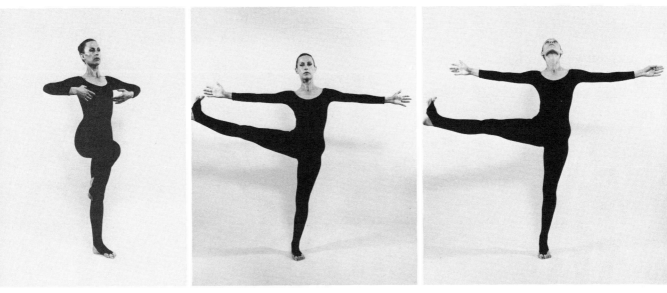

To the side, the working leg passes from parallel to turned-out passé on the 3-4, and is extended to the side (turned out) on 5-8. Then balance.

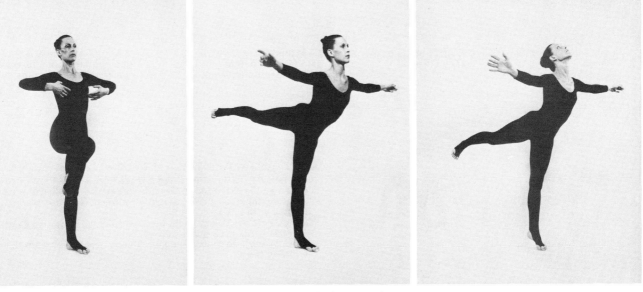

To the back, the working leg is parallel, both in the passé and in the extension.

This is a good exercise with which to build strength in the legs and control when standing on one leg. The contraction is an added complication which brings your entire body into play as you work for balance and control. Actually, it also strengthens your total body and improves your concentration. Always do it slowly. Remember, when doing the contraction and the movement to the back, to keep your body—as much as possible—in a classical arabesque position.—MM.

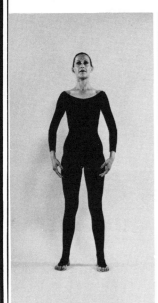

START in 1pp, arms down.

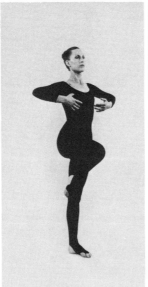

1-2 Lift R leg to passé parallel. Arms 1p.

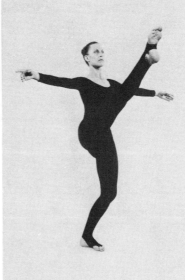

3-4 Extend R leg forward parallel with pointed foot and L leg in demi-plié. Arms 2p.

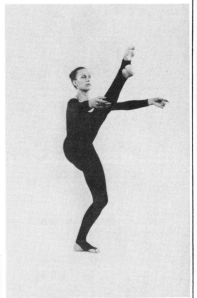

5-8 Contract forward over R leg and take arms forward parallel to floor, palms in.

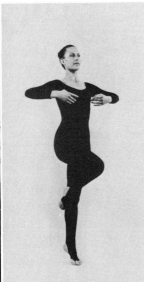

**1 Lift heel on bent L leg.
2-4 Hold and enlarge position.
5-6 Stretch L leg. Pull in R leg to passé parallel on balance. Arms 1p.**

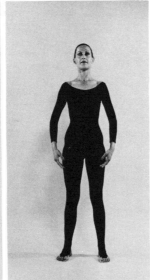

7-8 Lower arms and heel as you place R leg down in 1pp. Repeat from START with L leg.

DO THE EXERCISE WITH ALTERNATING LEGS EN CROIX:
(Left, below): To the side, R leg passes from parallel to turned-out passé and is extended to the side turned out on 3-4. Contract R side, stretch arms to R (L slightly rounded), towards working leg. Repeat with L leg.
(Center, below): To the back, the working leg is parallel. Contract forward and stretch arms down, palms in.
(Right, below): To the side, again, you contract *away* from the working leg.

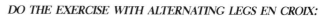

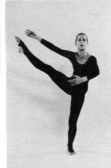

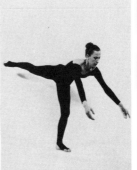

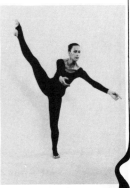

21. Lift and Flex, Bend and Point

A good exercise for building strength in your legs, this sequence will also improve your ability to go from point to flex and back to point. In order to develop strength in your legs, your leg muscles must go to the most extreme contracted position. When you point your foot in the air, on the floor, or at the side of your knee in the passé position, the calf muscle particularly must be in contraction.

Note: When your arms are up—or in second position—they should always reach to infinity.—MM.

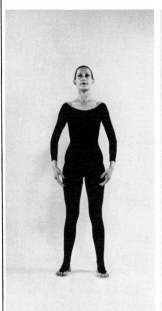 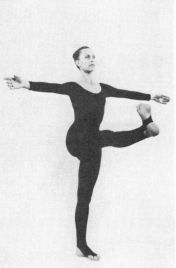 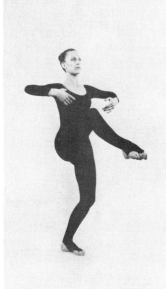 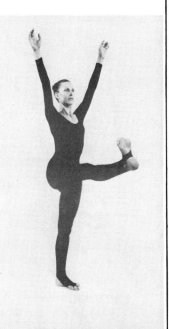

START in 1pp, arms down.

1 Push R leg sharply forward parallel with flexed foot. Arms 2p.
2-4 Hold and enlarge position.

5 Demi-plié softly on L leg and bend R to parallel forward attitude with pointed foot. Arms to 1p.
6-8 Hold and enlarge position.

1 Stretch L leg sharply and R leg forward, flexed foot. Arms up, palms forward.
2-4 Hold and enlarge position.

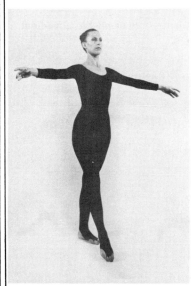 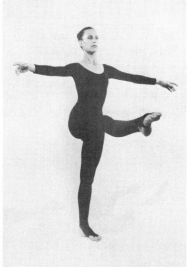 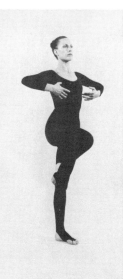 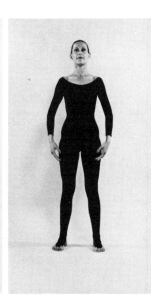

5 With sharp movement, place R leg parallel on floor in front, pointed foot. Arms 2p.

6 Lift R leg forward parallel with pointed foot.

7 Pull in R leg to passé parallel. Arms 1p.

8 Close R leg in 1pp and lower arms. Do exercise with alternating legs en croix. 63

Do exercise with alternating legs en croix:

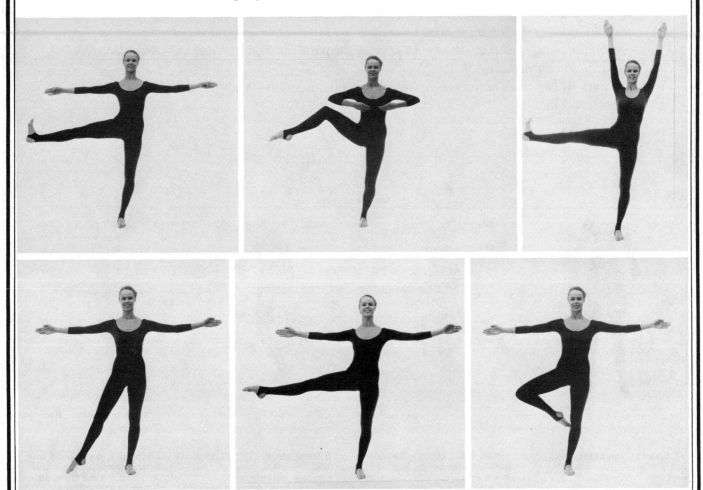

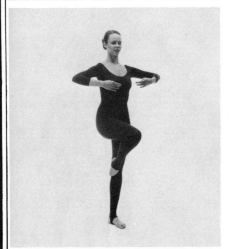

To the side, the turned-out working leg goes through passé turned-out to passé parallel and back to starting position.

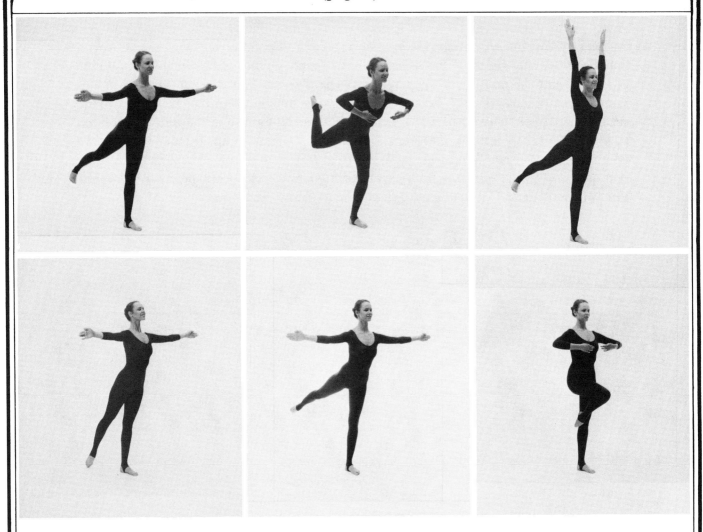

To the back, working leg is parallel.

Used in classical dance to develop the long leg line and well-pointed foot, this exercise is even more helpful as a leg isolation. In the grand rond de jambe in the air, be sure to maintain the center line and the position of the pelvis. Lift your torso as high away from the pelvis as possible while you pass through second position, and be sure not to lean too far forward in the arabesque (page 66, count 5-6). Many dancers lean too far forward in the next position too (page 67, count 7-8). Actually, the reverse is needed. Lift your body up and back while, at the same time, you lift and bend your back leg up as high as possible. When you twist your shoulders, don't move your arms from second position. Lock into second position and simply turn both shoulders. The standing leg should be in demi-plié throughout.—MM.

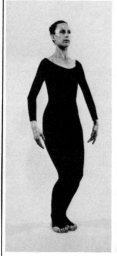 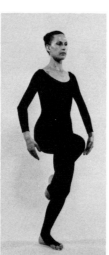 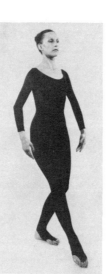 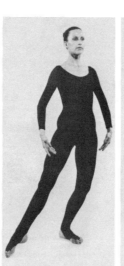 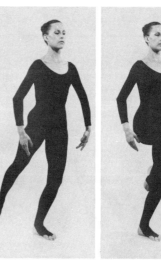

START in 1pp, demi-plié, arms rounded and down.

En dehors AND Lift R leg to passé parallel.

1-3 Rond de jambe a terre en dehors with R leg.

Leg should be parallel when in forward or back position. When out to the side, it should be turned out.

4 Pull in R leg to passé parallel. 5-8 Repeat from beginning.

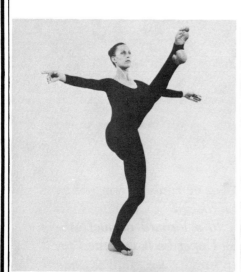 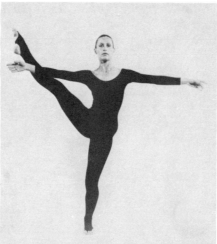 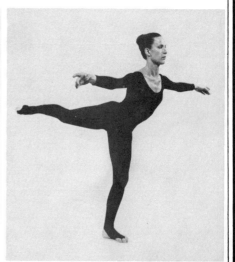

1-2 Stretch R leg forward parallel. Arms 2p.

3-4 Take R leg to side, turned out.

5-6 Take R leg to back parallel.

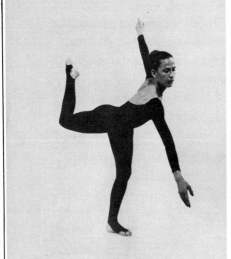 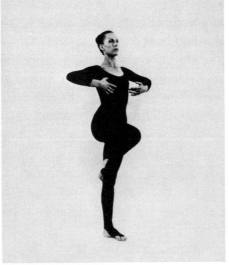 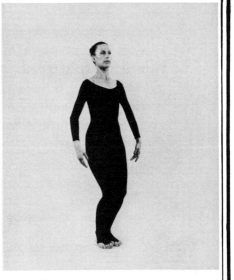

7-8 Bend leg to back parallel attitude. Upper body slightly forward, twist it to L. This places R arm diagonally down, L arm up, parallel to R lower leg.

1 Lift heel in demi-plié.
2-4 Hold balance.
5 Upper body to C. Stretch leg, lower heel, and pull in R leg to passé parallel. Arms 1p.
6 Hold and enlarge position.

7 Close R leg in 1pp demi-plié. Lower arms.
8 Enlarge position.
Repeat to other side.

Repeat with right and left leg en dedans.

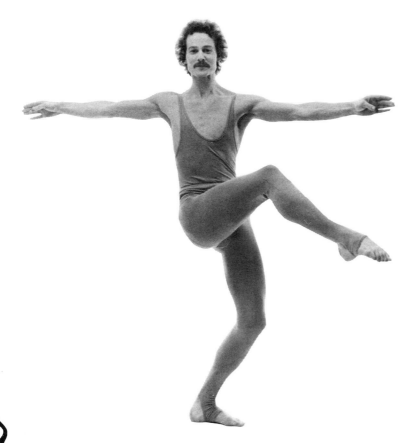

In ronds de jambe à terre and en l'air en dedans, the working leg is bent to a forward parallel attitude. Upper body is twisted towards working leg. Arms are then in 2p, one pointing directly forward and the other directly back.

This exercise was developed for coordination, to improve the reflex action of the leg movement from straight to bent and back to straight, and to improve the balance on half toe (which builds up the arch of the foot). It is done rapidly, especially by accomplished dancers. There are many versions of this exercise. Here the body is held in a steady position while leg and arm movements are isolated. Note that the leg movement comes from the knee and the arm action from the elbow on AND *2. This action is accented by leg, foot and arms.*

—MM.

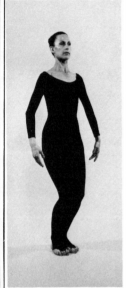 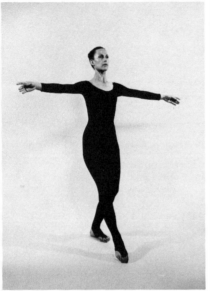 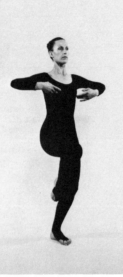 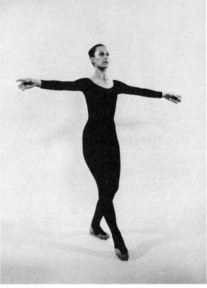

START in 1pp demi-plié, arms down.

1 Stretch R leg forward parallel on floor, arms to 2p.

AND Pull in R leg to passé parallel, arms to 1p.

2 Stretch R leg forward parallel on floor. Arms to 2p.

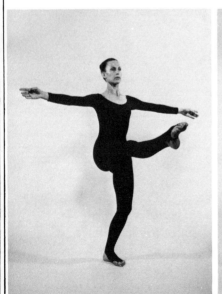 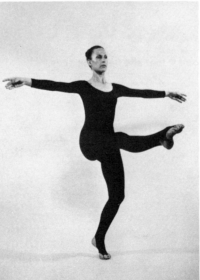 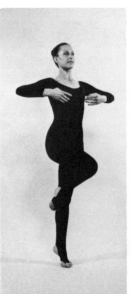 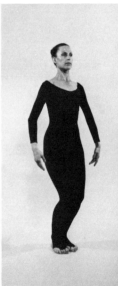

3 Close R leg in 1pp and lower arms.
4 Flick R leg forward parallel. Arms to 2p (above).

5 Lift L heel, staying in plié.
6 Hold and enlarge position.

7 Stretch L leg on half toe and pull in R to passé parallel. Arms to 1p.

8 Close R leg in 1pp demi-plié and lower arms. Do exercise en croix.

Designed to build control and balance in an off-center position, this exercise will also develop strength in the legs, if it is done regularly. Be sure to hold your body in a locked position—back absolutely flat—after your leg goes into second position.—MM.

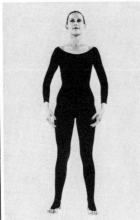

START in 1pp, arms down.

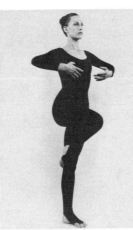

1 Lift **R** leg sharply to passé parallel. Arms to 1p.

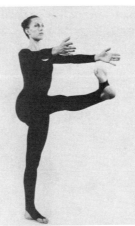

2 Extend **R** leg forward with flexed foot, arms forward parallel to floor, palms in.

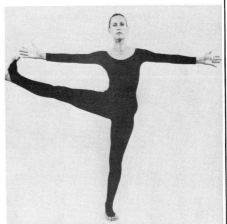

3-4 Take **R** leg to side turned out. Arms to 2p.

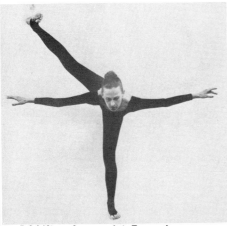

5-8 Lift up from waist. Expand as you take upper body forward at 90° angle with straight back (above). Turn **R** leg to parallel.

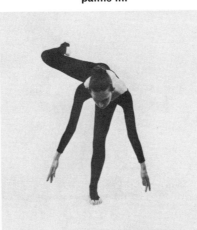

Point **R** foot and bend the knee 90° while lifting under **R** thigh (still to side) and demi-plié on **L** leg. Lower arms with palms facing each other.

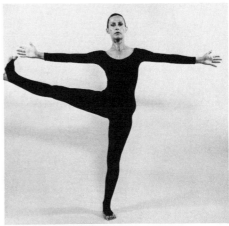

1 Lift **L** heel, in plié.
2-4 Hold and enlarge position.
5 Upper body C. Straighten **L** leg, lower heel. Turn hip under. Stretch **R** leg to side, flexed foot. Arms through 1p to 2p.

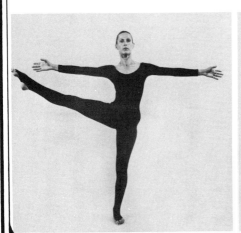

6 Point **R** foot.

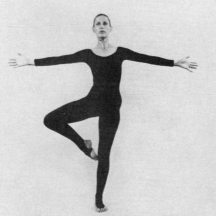

AND Pull in **R** leg to passé turned out (above).
7 Close **R** leg in passé parallel.

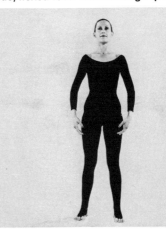

Arms to 1p.
8 Place **R** leg down in 1pp. Lower arms (above). Repeat to other side.

Remember here that your body and arms go in one direction, while your leg goes the opposite way. The front of your body must remain in a flat, open position—the way it would be if you were simply standing facing front. Don't allow your pelvis to push backwards so that you end up in a sway-back position. Control and balance as you turn your leg in the air, return it to a turned-out position, and return the pelvis to center.—MM.

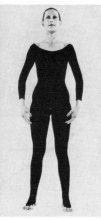
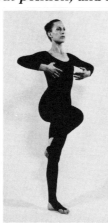
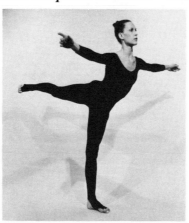
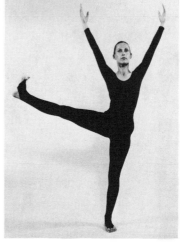

3-4 Take R leg to side, turned out. Stretch arms up, palms in.

START in 1pp, arms down.

1 Lift leg sharply to passé parallel. Arms to 1p.

2 Extend R leg back parallel with flexed foot. Arms to 2p.

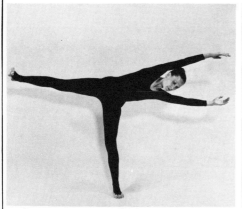
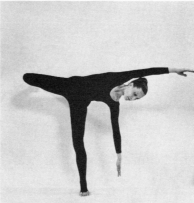
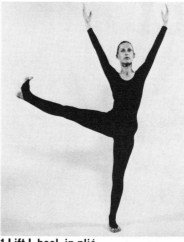

5-8 Lift from waist and expand as you take upper body to L. Turn R leg to parallel. Feel pull of arms and legs in opposite directions.

Point R foot and bend the knee 90° so that lower leg is invisible from front. Lift under R thigh (still to side) and demi-plié on L leg. Stretch L arm straight down, palm in.

**1 Lift L heel, in plié.
2-4 Hold and enlarge position.
5 Upper body to C. Straighten L leg and lower the heel. Turn hip under and turn out and stretch R leg to side, flexed foot. Arms up, palms in (above).**

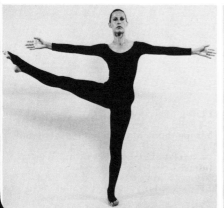
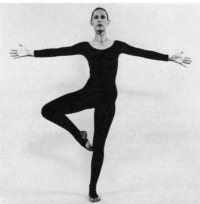
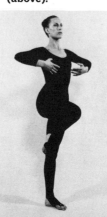
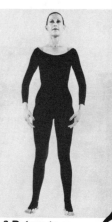

6 Point R foot. Arms to 2p.

AND Pull R leg in to passé, turned out.

7 R leg to passé parallel. Arms to 1p.

8 Return to START. Repeat to other side.

Another exercise that develops strength and control. When you do the layout to the back, pay special attention to the backwards arch and hold your chest well up. The strain of bending backward should not fall in the lumbar region, but instead in an arch high up under the shoulder blades. After the bend, be sure to return to an upright, standing position. Many students tend to leave the return unfinished, because of the bend.—MM.

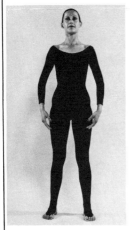
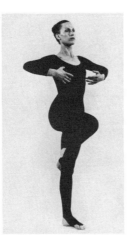
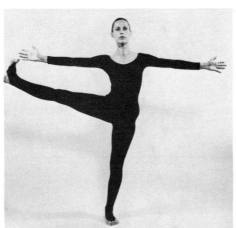
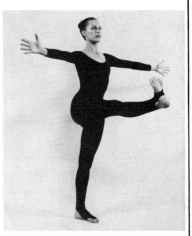

START in 1pp, arms down.

1 Lift **R** leg sharply to passé parallel. Arms to 1p.

2 Stretch **R** leg to side turned out, flexed foot. Arms to 2p.

3-4 Take **R** leg to front parallel.

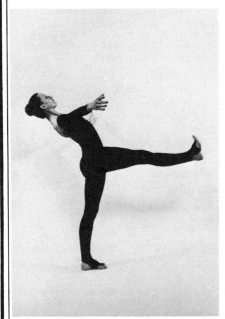
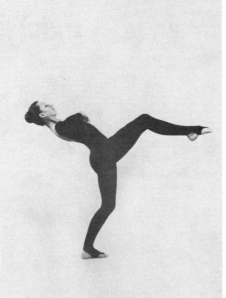
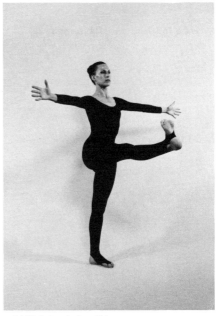

5-8 Lift up from waist and expand as you bend back (keep looking front).

Bend **R** leg to forward attitude parallel with pointed foot and demi-plié on **L** leg. Hold your **C** and take arms to 1p.

1 Lift **L** heel, in plié.
2-4 Hold and enlarge position.
5 Upper body to **C**, straighten **L** leg and lower the heel. Stretch **R** leg forward parallel with flexed foot. Arms to 2p (above).
6 Point **R** foot.
7 Pull in **R** leg to passé parallel. Arms to 1p.
8 Close **R** leg in 1pp and lower arms.

Repeat from START *to other side.*

Developed to improve the way you carry your body in a demi-plié, this exercise is also a good stretch for the muscles at the back of the kicking leg. That's the reason why the foot is flexed in the air. When you cross one foot underneath the other in the back, be careful not to push with that foot. The foot in the back is there only as a stabilizer; it's not to be used except to hold the Center.—MM.

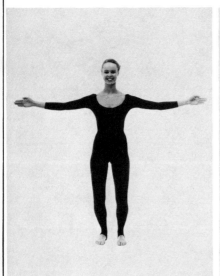 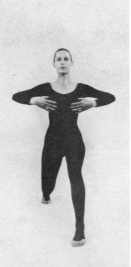 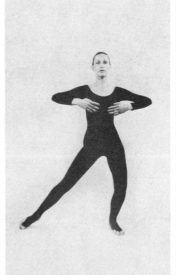 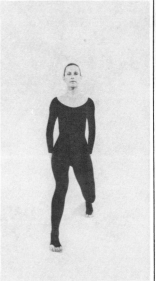

PART 1:
START in 1pp, demi-plié, arms in 2p.

1 Step R leg back in plié. Arms to 1p. AND Pull L leg to 1pp on ball of foot without weight.

2 Step L leg to wide 2 pp in plié (above). AND Pull in R leg to 1pp on ball of foot without weight.

3 Step R leg straight forward in plié and let arms fall behind back (above).

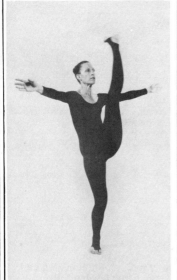 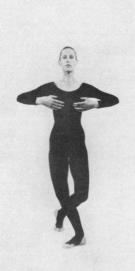 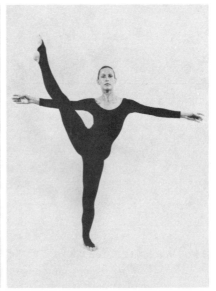

4 Kick L leg forward parallel with flexed foot and R leg in demi-plié. Arms to 2p. Accent.

5 Place L foot on ball under R leg, both slightly turned out. Place weight on L leg. Lower heel. Arms to 1p.

6 Flick R leg to side, turned out, with L leg in demi-plié. Arms to 2p. Accent (above). AND Close R leg in 1pp demi-plié.

7 Open to 2pp demi-plié. Let arms fall behind back.

8 Close both legs to 1pp demi-plié. Arms to 2p.

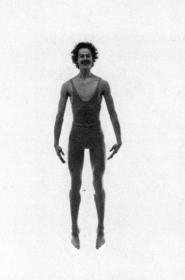

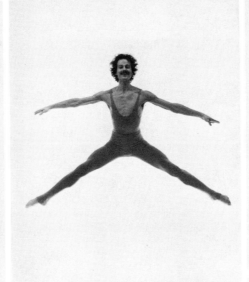

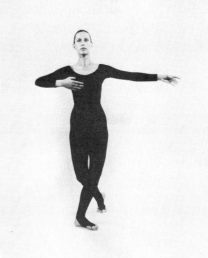

1–3 3 jumps in 1pp, arms down.
On 3: arms to 1p.

AND 4 Split-jump to 2pp and land in 1pp.
Arms to 2pp, palms down in the jump.
5–8 Repeat last 4 counts.

AND 1 Shift weight R/L: Step R leg bent to R and step L across, both slightly turned out. R arm to 1p and L to 2p.
2 Hold and enlarge position.
3–4 Stretch R arm to L diagonally forward parallel to floor. Twist upper body slightly to L.

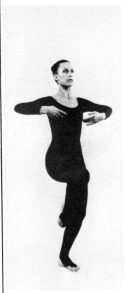

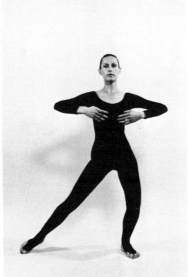

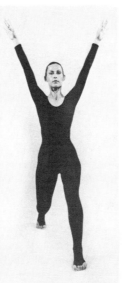

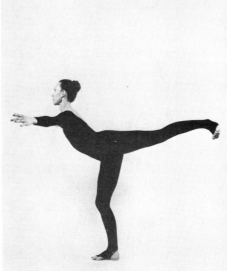

5-7 Turn en dehors to R with R leg in passé parallel. To start the turn, open R arm quickly to 2p, then close both arms to 1p.
8 Close R leg in 1pp and lower arms. Repeat PART 1 to other side.

PART 2:
1 Step R leg straight forward in pliè. Arms to 1p.
AND Pull in L leg to 1pp on ball of foot without weight.
2 Step L leg to wide 2pp in plié (above).
AND Pull in R leg to 1pp on ball of foot without weight.

3 Step R leg straight back in plié and stretch arms up, palms forward.

4 Kick L leg back parallel with flexed foot and R leg in demi-plié. Arms to 2p. Accent.

Continue as in PART 1 with flick to side, jumps and turns.

Repeat from beginning of PART 2 to other side.

On facing page: Matt Mattox and Annette Plottin

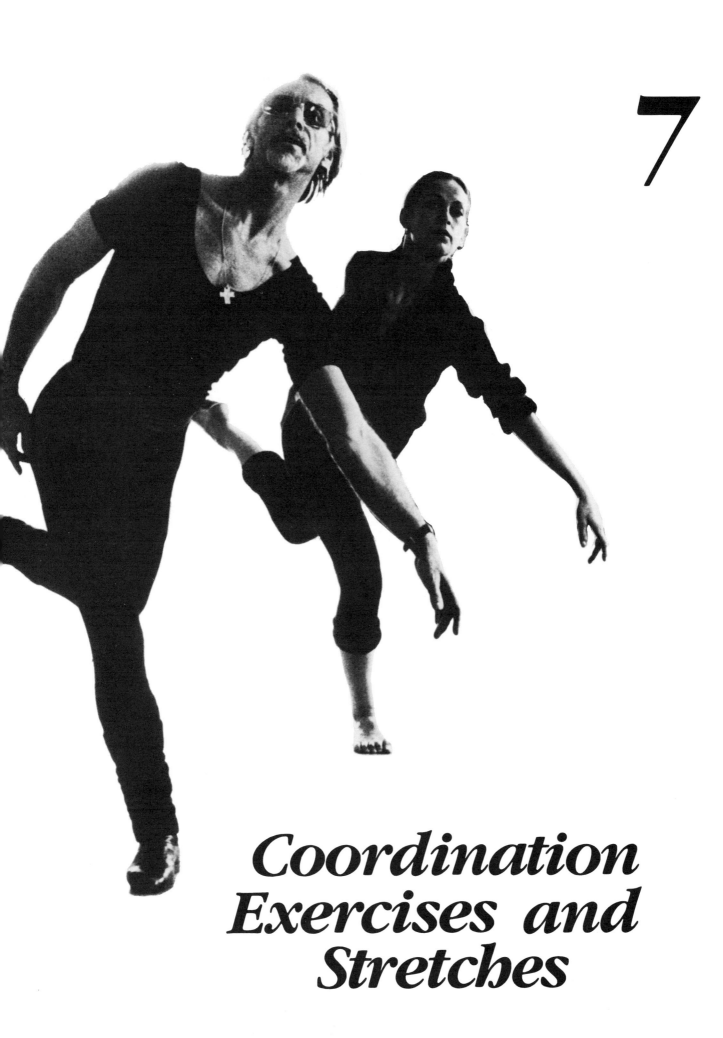

7

Coordination Exercises and Stretches

An excellent exercise for coordination, this one is easy to do slowly, though it's hard on arm and shoulder muscles. It's extremely difficult to do it quickly, however: the problems are in concentration. The turned-in and turned-out positions are equally important. To turn hands in, put palms back. When hands are turned out, palms are forward.—MM.

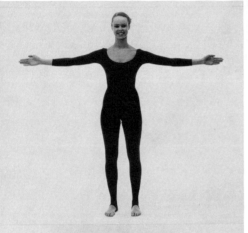

START in 1pp, arms in 2p.

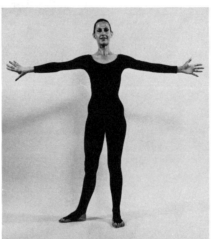

PART 1:
AND Turn in R hand.
1 Place R leg in 2p, turned out.

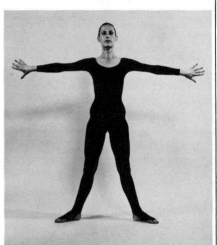

AND Turn in L hand.
2 Place L leg in 2p, turned out.

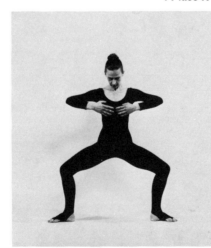

3 Grand plié and let head fall forward. Arms to 1p.

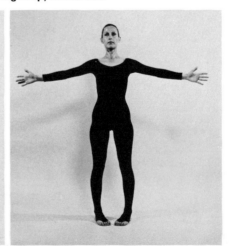

4 Close legs in 1p turned in. Head to C, arms to 2p, turned out.
5-8 Repeat from the beginning 3 times.

ON TO PART 2

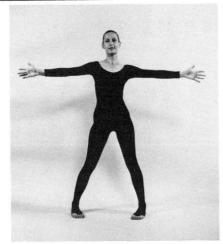

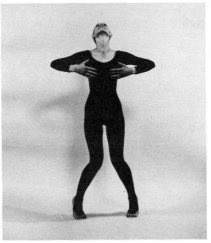

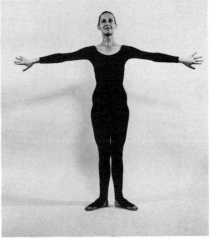

PART 2:
Keep hands in position and continue:
1 Place R leg in 2p, turned in.
2. Place L leg in a wide 2p, turned in.

3 Bend knees and lift heels while lifting head back. Arms to 1p.

4 Close legs in 1p, turned out with straight knees. Turn in both hands (above).
AND Turn out R hand.

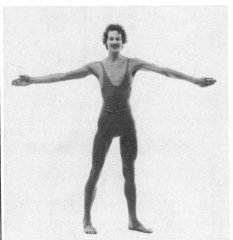

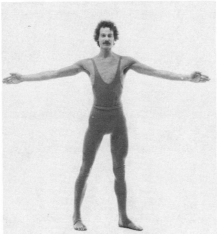

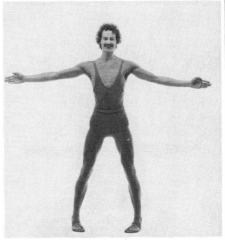

5 Place R leg in 2p turned in.

AND Turn out L hand.

6 Place L leg in 2p, turned in.

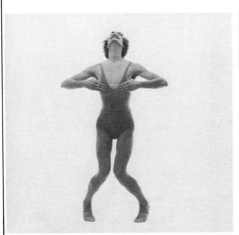

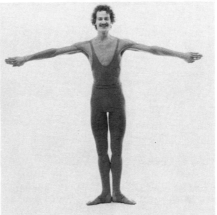

7 Bend knees and lift heels while lifting head back. Arms to 1p.

8 Close legs in 1p, turned out, with straight knees. Turn in both hands (above).
Repeat AND 5-8, twice.

Keep position in hands and repeat from PART 1 to other side.

Exactly as was the previous exercise, this one is easy slow, but not so easy fast. Excellent for coordination.

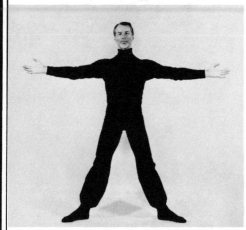

START in 2p, turned out, arms in 2p.

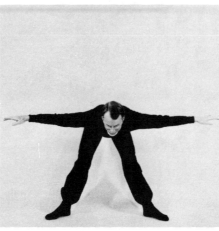

1 Lift up from waist. Take upper body forward at 90° angle with straight back.

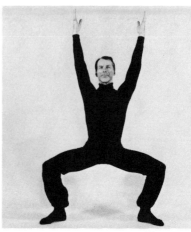

2 Grand plié and upper body to **C**. Stretch arms up, palms in.

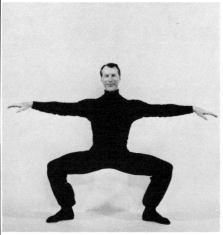

3 Arms to 2p, palms down.

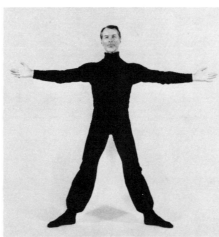

4 Straighten knees and turn palms forward.

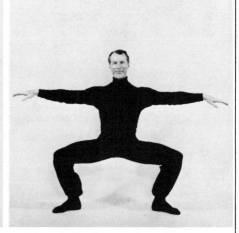

5 Grand plié. Arms to 2p, palms down.

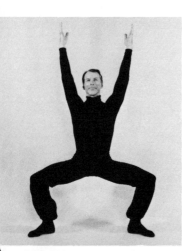

6 Stretch arms up, palms in.

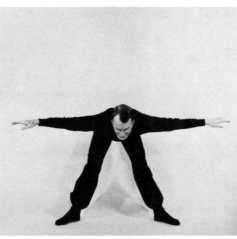

7 Take upper body forward at 90° angle with straight back and straighten knees. Arms to 2p, palms down.

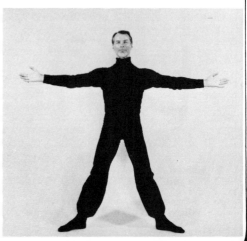

8 Upper body to **C**, arms in 2p. Repeat several times.

Similar to the two previous exercises, this sequence will improve your coordination. The more coordination exercises you do, the sooner you'll be able to think rapidly—essential when you dance a routine.—MM.

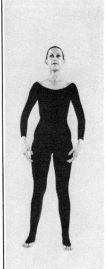

START in 1pp, arms down.

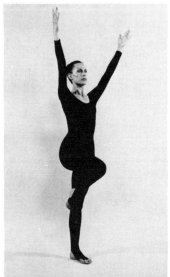

PART 1:
1 Lift R leg to passé parallel. Stretch arms forward and up, palms in.

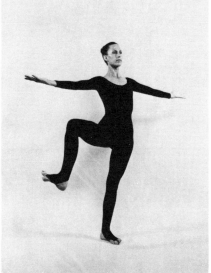

2 Turn out R leg to side; hip and knee should be at 90° angle, flexed foot. Arms to 2p, palms up.

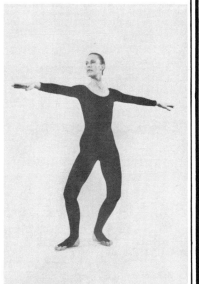

AND turn palms down.
3 Place R leg down in 2p turned out with L leg in demi-plié (above). Turn head to R.

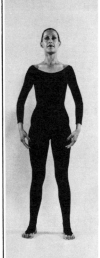

4 Straighten knees as you pull in R leg to 1pp. Lower arms. Head to C.
5-8 Repeat PART 1 to L, but turn head to R.

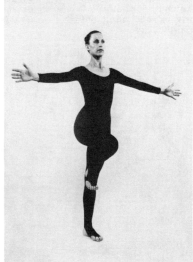

PART 2:
1 Lift R leg to passé parallel with flexed foot. Arms to 2p.

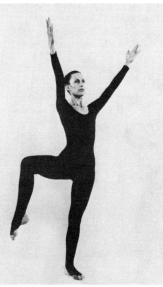

2 Turn out R leg to side, pointed foot. Stretch arms up, palms in.

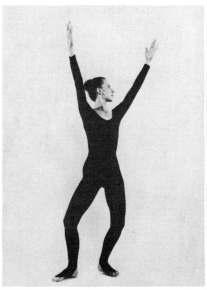

3 Place R leg down in 2p, turned out, L leg in demi-plié. Turn head to L.
4 Straighten knees as you pull in R leg to 1pp. Arms to 2p, palms down, head C.
5-8 Repeat last 4 counts to L, but turn head to L.
1-8 Repeat PART 2 to R and L.

This stretch exercise is good for the backs of your legs, good for the holding of the body in a straight-back position, and good for using the body totally. Remember that, in all the stretches to the front, the stretch happens because the back is held straight at the same time that you bend forward from the hip socket—not from the top of the pelvis. Bending from the top of the pelvis results in a round-back position, and with the back rounded, the stretch is minimal. One more point: don't let your elbow touch your knee while bending to the side.

—MM.

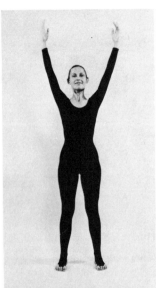

START in 1pp, arms down.

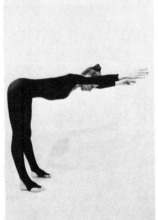

1 Stretch both arms forward and up, palms in.

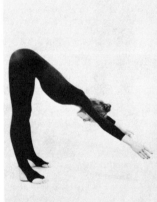

2 Lift up from waist and stretch upper body forward at 90° angle with straight back.

3 Stretch upper body down at 45° angle with straight back.

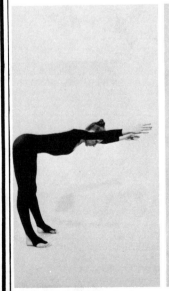

4 Stretch upper body forward

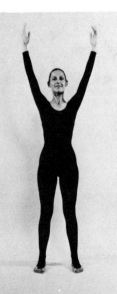

and again to C, arms overhead.

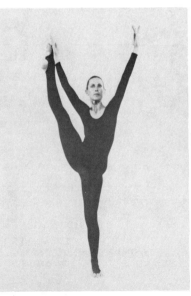

5 Kick R leg to 2p, turned out, with force.
6 Place R leg down in 2pp, leaving arms up.

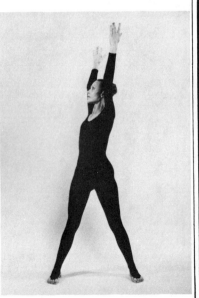

7 Twist upper body to R, keeping pelvis still.

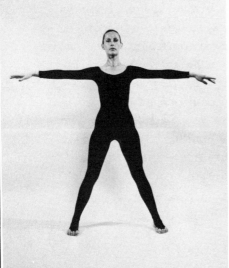

8 Upper body to C, arms to 2p, palms down.

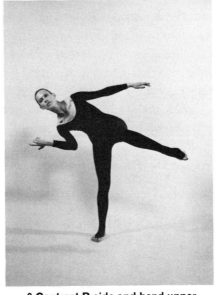

9 Contract R side and bend upper body to R. Fold R arm. Push elbow to L in front of chest. Fold L leg underneath you at an angle just under 90° between thigh and lower leg. Accent.

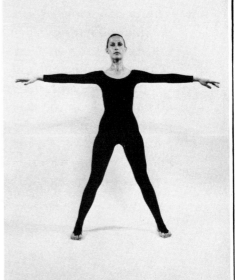

AND Place L leg in 2pp. Arms to 2p, palms down (above).

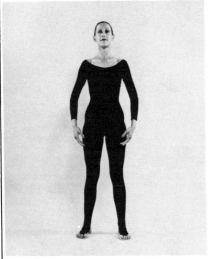

10 Close R leg in 1pp and lower arms.

Repeat from the beginning to the other side.

32. Fall Forward + Bounce and Stretch

This exercise loosens the backs of the legs and calls for a quick reaction as the body bends to the side and returns to a full standing position. From both the forward bend and the one to the side, be sure you return to the full standing position with buttocks contracted. Don't cut corners in standing up fully before you continue to the next part of the exercise.

The bounce and stretch is also good for the backs of the legs, and the walk forward—keeping heels on the floor—extends the stretch. The contraction and release extends the stretch even more. In the contraction, the hamstring muscle is relaxed a bit, but in the released position, it is used totally. This exercise is also good for learning to use the back fluently, starting with the sacroiliac and moving down or—if you prefer—up to the head, vertebra by vertebra.—MM.

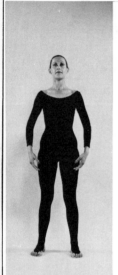 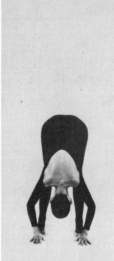 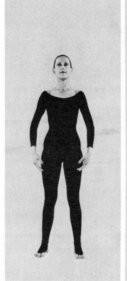 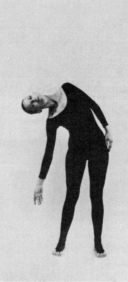 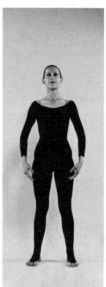

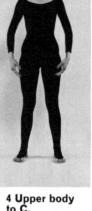

START in 1pp, arms down.

PART 1:
1 Let upper body fall forward, palms touching floor.

2 Upper body to **C**, bouncing back up with a straight back.

3 Let upper body fall to R. R arm stretches toward floor.

4 Upper body to **C**.
5-8 Repeat from **START** to other side.

Repeat this exercise several times.

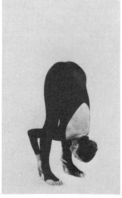

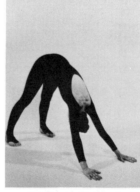 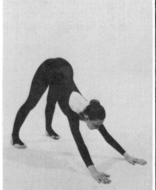

PART 2:
Bend knees completely, heels off floor. Relax upper body forward; place palms on floor. Bounce once.

2 AND 3 Repeat bounce 3 times (make 2 bounces slow and 2 fast).
4 (above) Lower heels and straighten knees with straight back.

Take hold around outside of ankles and pull upper body to thighs.
___
Repeat from the beginning of PART 2 several times.
___
PART 3:
1-4 Release back and hips and walk forward on hands—R/L/R/L—as far as you can with heels on floor, lifting head.

5-8 Contract, bend head under. Place weight forward into arms (above).

1-4 Release, lift head and place weight back into legs (right above).
5-8 Repeat 5-8.

1-4 Repeat 1-4.
5-8 Hold release and "walk" hands towards legs.
1-8 Roll up through spine—vertebra by vertebra—to standing position.

82

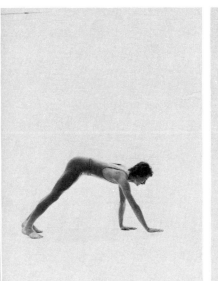
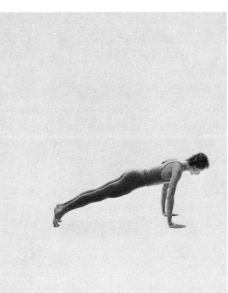
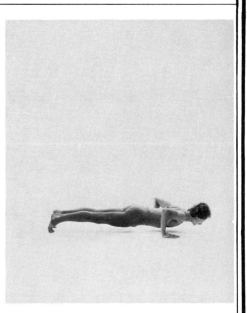

VARIATION: After last release in PART 3, lift heels, continue to "walk" hands forward to prone position and do push-ups.

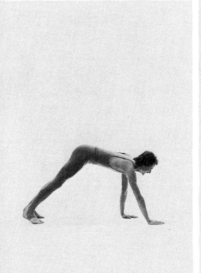
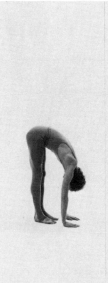
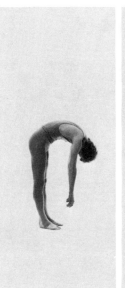
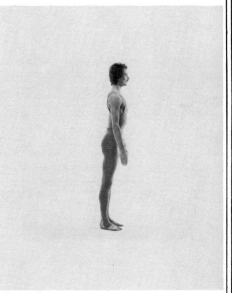

Walk back on hands towards legs and roll up vertebra by vertebra to standing position.

On facing page: Matt Mattox and Elisabeth Frich

8

Floor Exercises

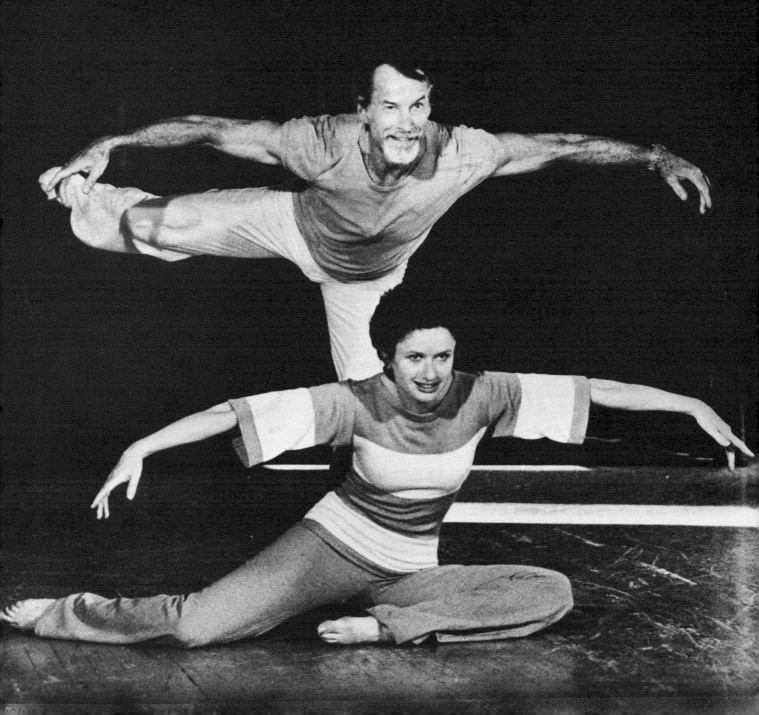

This exercise is designed for stretching around the hip socket, while you sit on the floor. Turning against your leg—at the same time that you pull on your knee—creates a stretch on the exterior side of the hip. Your buttocks must be on the floor. After returning to a relaxed position, carrying your leg to the back creates a different kind of strength in the working muscles. When you place your leg on the floor parallel and straight—and take your body backwards—the front of your hip should be opened and stretched as much as possible. At the same time, keep the opposite buttock resting on the floor (right leg back/left buttock on floor). This creates an exterior stretch on the sitting side, and also in front of the working hip. When you return to your original position, take hold of the leg that's in the air (preferably on the heel) and pull it towards you (keep it well turned out). This develops the back muscles which help you sustain a sitting position when the leg is relaxed. Move your head back to help you lift your chest and hold the position before continuing the exercise.

When you change from one side to the other, hold your back rigidly straight and use your legs in isolation, arms stretched to infinity.—MM.

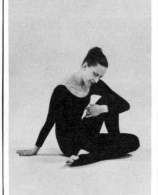
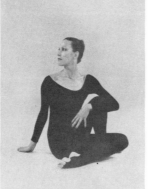
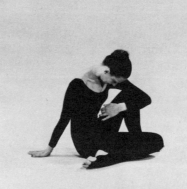
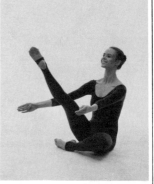

START by sitting on both hips, **R** leg bent over **L**, and **R** foot as close to **L** hip as possible. Support with **R** arm behind **R** hip. Point **L** foot. Wrap **L** arm around **R** knee. Relax upper body forward.

PART 1:
1-4 Stretch up from lower back, turning to **R**, holding **C**. Pull **R** thigh into body with **L** arm. Breathe in.

5-8 Relax upper body forward and breathe out.
Repeat **PART 1** several times.

PART 2:
1-4 Stretch **R** leg up, turned out, and upper body to **R** diagonal front, sitting on both hips. Arms forward to **R** diagonal front parallel to floor, palms in.

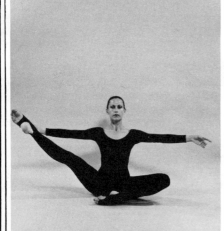
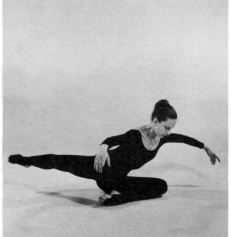
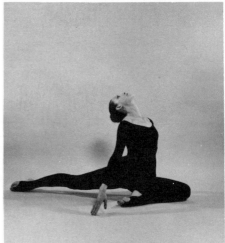

5-8 Take **R** leg to 2p (above), bending it to parallel attitude and

leaning slightly forward. Finish by placing **R** leg on floor in 4p. Arms to 2p, palms down.

1-8 Stretch **R** leg on floor to pt 6. Lift well up from waist and start bending back in upper body. Support with hands on floor.

33. Right Leg Over Left (page 2)

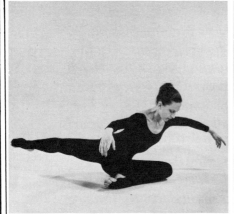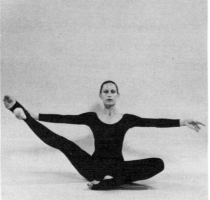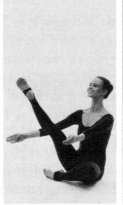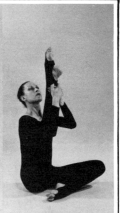

1-4 Finish backbend. Lean upper body slightly forward again and pull in R leg, carrying it to attitude side parallel. Arms to 2p.

5-8 Sit on both hips. Stretch R leg to side—

and carry it forward, turned out.

1-8 Take R ankle with both hands and pull in leg to chest 4 times, facing pt 2.

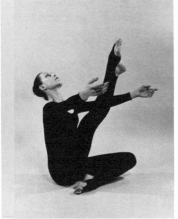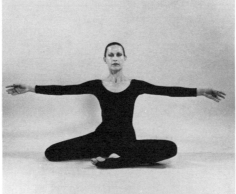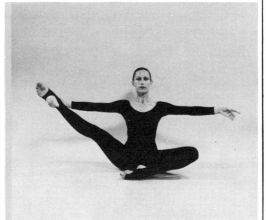

1-7 Let go of R leg and lift head back.
8 Place R leg bent over L in starting position.

Repeat PART 2 several times. The last time, place R leg behind in 4p (above) on floor. Change to other side.

PART 3:
1-2 Stretch R leg turned out to side in air.

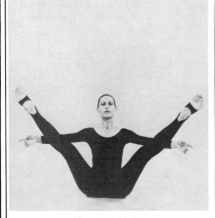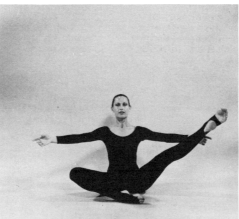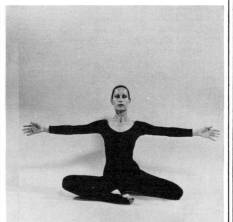

Then add L leg.

3 Bend R leg on floor in front.

4 Bend L leg on floor behind in 4p.

Repeat change 2 times, finishing with L leg over R to start from PART 1 to the other side.

This exercise is designed to loosen up the leg and hip socket. Start with both hips down. When you move your hip up, stretch open as much as possible. When you replace your hip, try to put it back down to the floor so that you're sitting on both buttocks. When you stretch to the right or left, open the leg opposite to the stretch and use your foot to help you push your body into its most stretched position. While stretching, keep your spine in a straight line. Bend directly to the side, not to the front or back. Many students allow themselves to "lean" forward or back, without realizing they're doing it.

In the last part of the stretch, you'll be continuing to work on loosening the hamstring. The roll to the back while you're lying on the floor is designed to open the front of your hip as well as stretch the long thigh muscles in the front of your leg. Many students find that the working knee (the knee of the leg that is bent to the back) wants to come up in the air as you arrive on your back. Push it back down as soon as you can.

It is vitally important to relax, blow the air out of your body, and get your back (totally on the floor) in a direct line—a normal position, as if you're standing or sitting. Don't let your spine make a curve while you're on your back.—MM.

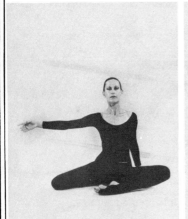
START by sitting on both hips in 4p, R leg bent behind and L leg bent in front. R arm 2p, L on floor behind you.

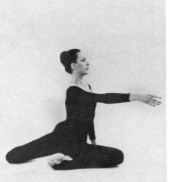
PART 1:
1-4 Tighten buttocks on R side and push hip forward and up. Turn upper body to L. Stretch R arm forward and to L.

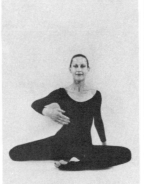
5-8 Lower R hip and return upper body to C. Round R arm in front of body and take it to 2p.

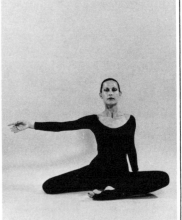
Keep lifting up from waist. Repeat **PART 1** several times.

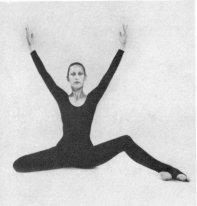
PART 2:
AND Place L leg to side, sole of foot turned out on floor. Arms to side and up, palms in.

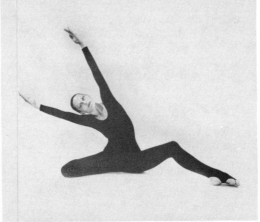
1-4 Lift up from waist, stretch up and to R. Keep spine aligned. Look in direction of hands.
5-8 Upper body to C, arms 2p, palms up. Repeat **PART 2** several times.

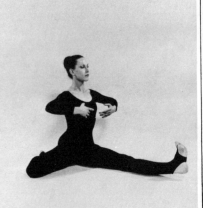
PART 3: Clean, crisp movements.
AND Stretch leg forward on floor to pt 1, flexed foot. Arms to 1p.

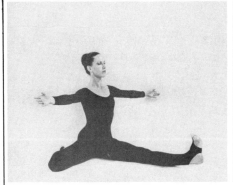

1 Arms to 2p.

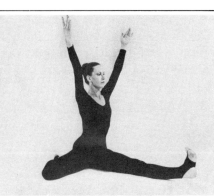

2 Stretch arms up, palms in.

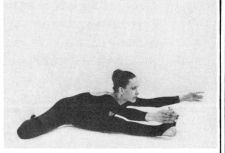

3 Stretch upper body forward with straight back, arms forward.

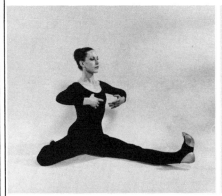

4 Upper body to C. Arms 1p. Repeat PART **3 several times. The last time, stop on count 3, take hold of L foot with both hands and stay down in**

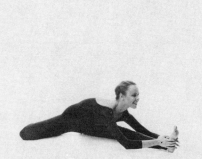

long stretch (above) for at least 8 counts. Then take upper body to C, arms to 1p.

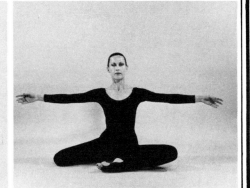

PART 4:
AND **Bend L leg on floor in front to 4p.**

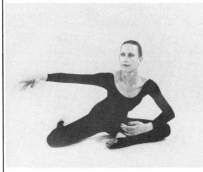

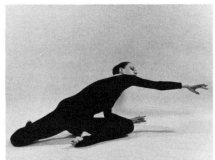

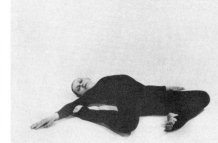

1-3 Swing upper body and arms to R. Place L hand on the floor behind L thigh to pt 5. Swing R arm in a big circle to L, then overhead and to R, as you lie on the floor.
4 Hold and enlarge position with arms in 2p, palms to floor, contracting to flatten back to floor.
5-8 Reverse swing action to come up to sitting position, arms in 2p. Repeat PART **4 several times.**
The last time: 1-4 as before.
5-8 Hold and enlarge position on floor. Then change to other side:

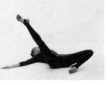

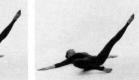

1-2 Stretch R and then L leg to side, turned out in air.

3 Bend R leg in front on floor.

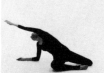

4 Bend L leg in back to 4p on floor.

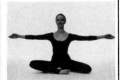

5-8 Push off with arms and reverse swing

action so you come up sitting in 4p, arms in 2p.

Repeat from PART *1 several times, alternating sides.*

35. 90 Degrees

Designed for achieving precision in feet and leg positions, this is also another good coordination exercise. You can make it into a stretch for the hamstring by grasping the back of the thigh of the leg that's in the air. Hold the knee against your chest while you do point and flex; then return to the starting position. If you use this exercise as a stretch, you won't derive any benefit from it for coordination, but if you use 4 slow counts, for point, point and flex, you'll find it very good for your legs.—MM.

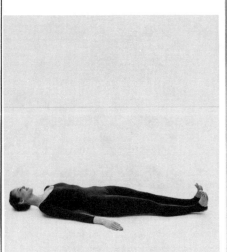

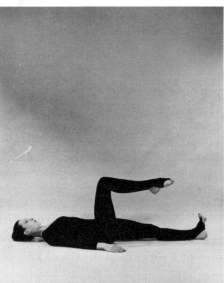

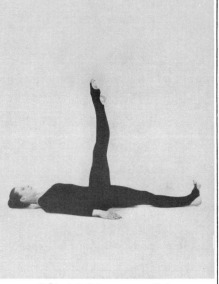

START by lying on your back with straight legs in pp, feet flexed and arms alongside, straight knees.

1 Bend **R** leg at 90° angle from hip to knee—and knee to foot. Lower leg is parallel to floor.

2 Stretch **R** leg up parallel.

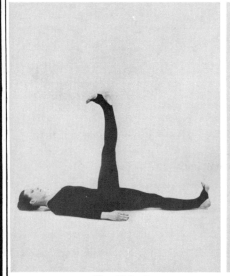

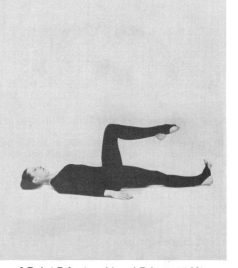

AND Flex **R** foot.

3 Point **R** foot and bend **R** knee at 90° angle.
4 Flex **R** foot and stretch **R** leg as you lower it forward to starting position.
5–8 Repeat from START.

Repeat several times with alternating legs.

This exercise is also good for warming up feet and ankles.

This exercise is good for the legs, the back and the stomach. By using the flex/point, you work the feet, and then the long, stretched leg. The stomach muscles are worked by using a slow, controlled roll up and down, contracting as you lift off the floor—one vertebra at a time—and lying back down the same way. There's also a stretch for the hamstring in this exercise—when you take the body as far forward and over the legs as possible before sitting up. It's important to sit up quickly on the count of 8, and to contract quickly on the count of 1, for the return to the floor.—MM.

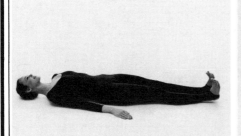

START by lying on your back, with straight legs in pp, feet flexed and arms alongside.

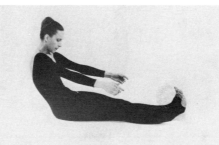

PART 1:
1-6 Lift head and shoulders and press lower back onto floor as you roll up vertebra by vertebra through

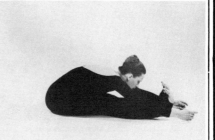

spine. Arms forward, palms in. Finish roll-up with upper body rounded forward (above).

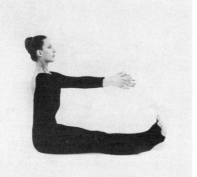

8 Straighten back as you take body to sitting position. Arms forward, palms in.

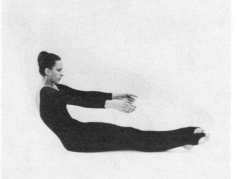

1 Point feet and contract pelvis.
2-7 Roll down to back, vertebra by vertebra.
8 Flex feet (above).

Repeat PART 1 several times.

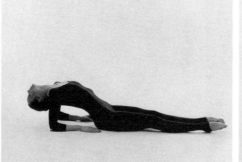

PART 2:
1-8 High arch, contracting back, lifting shoulders and head in air. Support yourself on elbows. Point feet.

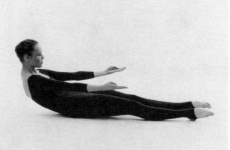

1-8 Contract pelvis under and roll down on back, vertebra by vertebra with arms in front of you.

Repeat PART 2 several times.

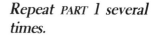

37. The Plow (Shoulder Stand)

This exercise is an excellent one for relaxing the neck and shoulder muscles, and it is also good for stretching the back totally. The more you can place the pelvis over your head, the more benefit you can get from this exercise. As you return to a prone position, replace your spine vertebra by vertebra as much as possible.—MM.

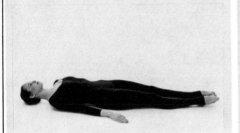

START by lying on your back with straight legs in pp, feet pointed and arms alongside. Straight knees, pointed feet.

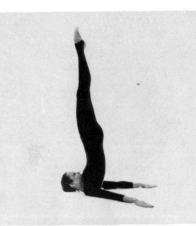

1-4 Lift legs parallel towards ceiling. Let hips lift as well.

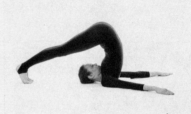

5-8 Extend legs overhead while taking weight onto shoulders. Flex feet as you place them on floor behind you.

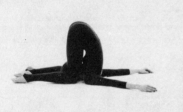

1-4 Point feet, bend knees and place them next to your ears and relax.

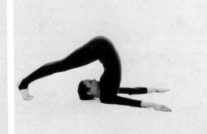

5-8 Straighten knees and flex feet.

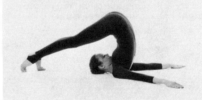

1-4 "Walk away" (from head) to pt 5 R/L/R/L, keeping legs straight.

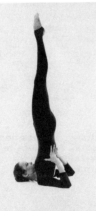

5-8 Lift legs up to ceiling with pointed feet. Support yourself with your hands, if necessary.

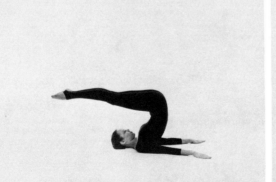

1-8 Roll down to starting position, vertebra by vertebra.

Repeat from the beginning several times.

Good for the stomach muscles, this exercise also helps develop control, as you lift your body into position with legs bent, keeping torso and legs working together. Be careful not to bring up the body separate from the legs. And don't change the back into a rounded position while you're putting your legs in a stretched position. When you return to the floor, your torso and legs should arrive simultaneously. You can do this in another way: after arriving in the straight-leg position, open your legs to second position (see last photo below), then return to the closed position—maintaining the straight back—before returning to the prone position.

—MM.

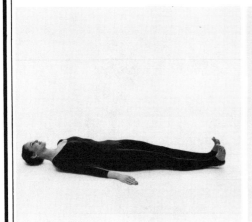

START by lying on your back, legs in pp, straight knees, flexed feet, arms alongside.

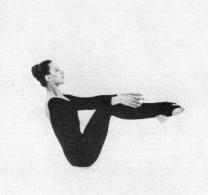

1 Bend knees and sit up with lower legs parallel to floor and pointed feet. Keep back straight. Arms parallel forward, palms in.

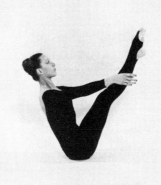

2-4 Hold and enlarge position.
5-8 (above) Stretch legs up parallel.

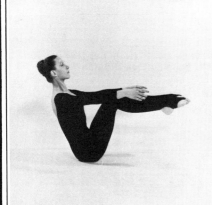

1 Bend knees.
2-4 Hold and enlarge position.

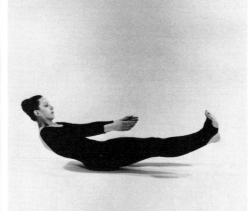

5-8 Simultaneously straighten knees, flex feet, contract pelvis under and lower your legs as you return to starting position.

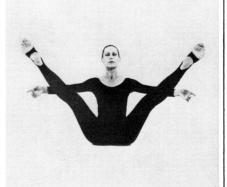

VARIATION:
After arriving at straight leg position (count 5, third picture), open legs to 2p (counts 6-7), then close them (count 8) and return to START.

Repeat from the beginning several times.

Here again is a stretch for the back of the legs while in a sitting position. There should be strong accent on the count of 3—at the moment of the forward stretch—as well as an expulsion of air from the lungs at the same time, which gives you the chance for a longer stretch. Keep your feet in a fixed position, so that you can stretch the hamstring as fully as possible.—MM.

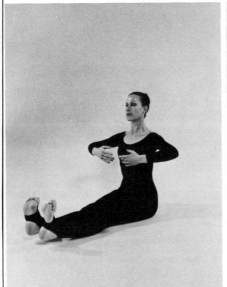

START by sitting in 1pp with flexed feet, arms in 1p.

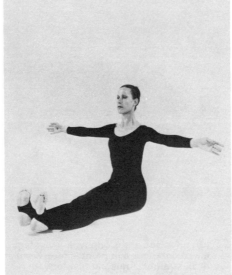

1 Arms to 2p.

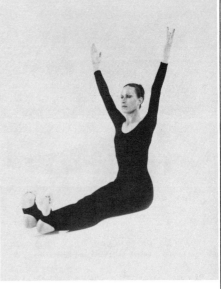

2 Lift up from waist and stretch arms up, palms in.

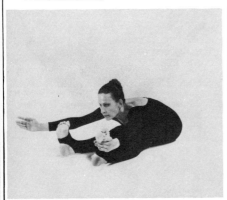

3 Stretch arms and upper body forward with straight back.

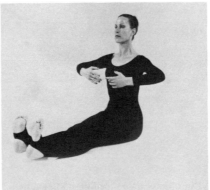

4 Return to START.
Repeat from beginning several times.

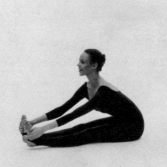

The last time: Stop on count 3. Take hold of feet (around the outsides) and stay down in long stretch (above). Then return to START.

Distinctly an exercise for the development of a very wide open second position. At the moment you lift the buttocks into the air, it is very important to relax the stretch as much as possible. Advanced students should try to work for the roll forward, finishing on the stomach. There's an advantage to doing several bend-and-stretch positions before rolling forward. Hold the body well forward, with the back straight, as you do those repeated stretches, to open second position as much as you can before continuing forward to the stomach.—MM.

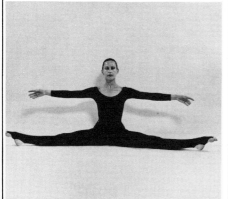

START in 2p turned out with pointed feet, arms in 2p.

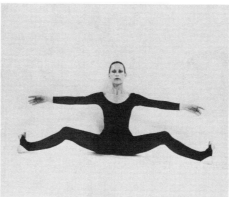

PART 1:
1-2 Bend knees and flex feet.

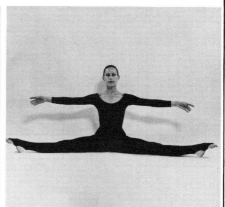

3-4 Straighten knees and point feet. Repeat **PART 1** several times.

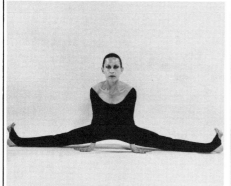

PART 2:
1-2 Place hands on floor in front—

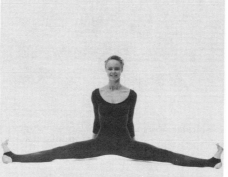

or in back of you, and take weight into arms.
3-4 Turn out and sit in wider 2p, as you point feet.

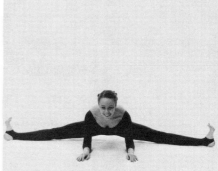

Repeat **PART 2** several times. The last time, pass body far enough forward so that you

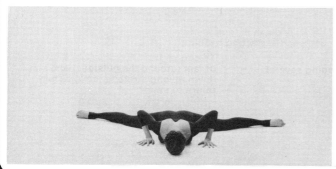

roll forward completely, turning legs in.

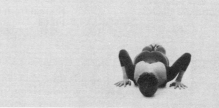

Close your legs as you finish on your stomach.

For same purpose as preceding exercise.—MM.

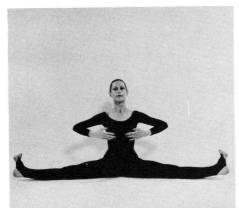

START by sitting in 2p turned out, with
flexed feet and arms in 1p.

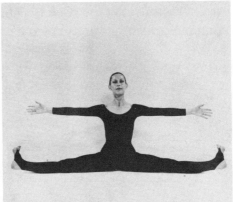

1 Arms to 2p.

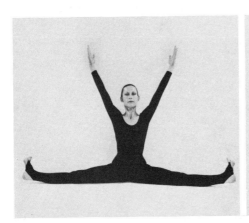

2 Lift up from waist and stretch arms up
with palms in.

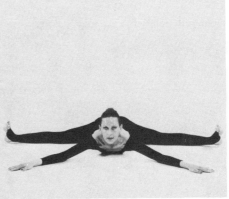

3 Stretch upper body forward with
straight back, keeping legs turned out.

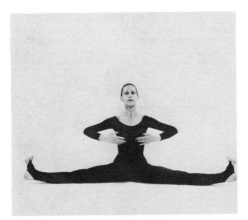

4 Return to starting position.
Repeat from beginning several times.

The last time, stop on count 3 and
stay down in long stretch. Then go
back to starting position.

This exercise (as well as the last two) is designed to loosen the hamstring, and the tendons and muscles at the interior part of the leg. In second position, it helps develop a good extension— above the level of the waist to the front and to the side. It's also good for developing a high kick to the front and side.—MM.

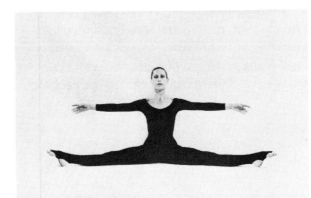

START by sitting in 2p, turned out with pointed feet, arms in 2p.

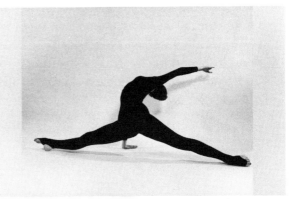

1-4 Take weight onto **R** hand on floor behind you as you lift pelvis and turn to **R**. Swing **L** arm in big circle down and towards **R** arm overhead and finish in high arch (above).
5-8 Split forward, taking **L** arm through 2p and to floor.

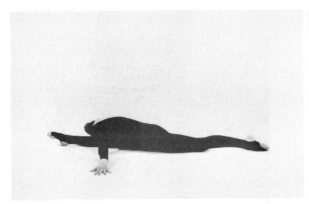

1-4 Lift up from waist and stretch forward over **R** leg.
5-8 Bend back, holding your center and return to **C**.

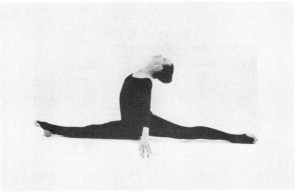

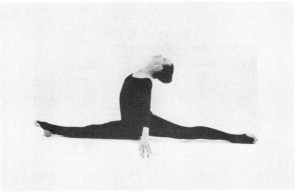

Repeat from the beginning several times, alternating sides.

1-4 Take weight onto **R** arm, swing **L** overhead and lift pelvis.
5-8 Turn pelvis to front. Sit in wider 2p, turned out, lifting **R** and lowering **L** arm to 2p.

This exercise usually starts with 4 kicks, while you lie on your stomach—R/L/R/L—after which you lift your body totally in the air. If you started with a kick from your R leg, you hold your right leg in the air and then simply walk backwards by using your hands, keeping the supporting foot in place. When you've arrived at a standing position on one leg, it's exactly the same as being in a split. There is one difference: it is possible to make even a bigger split by forcing the leg in the air further forward over the head. After the walk back, remember to hold the leg that's in the air as far over your head as possible as you return to the position on the floor, thus working the back actively for a good arabesque position. This exercise is very good for stretching the standing leg, strengthening the arms and developing strength in the back for the arabesque.—MM.

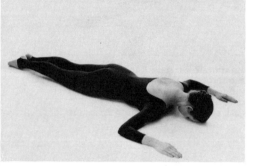

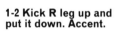

1-2 Kick R leg up and put it down. Accent.

3-8 Repeat kick with L/R/L leg.

START **by lying on your stomach with legs in pp and hands on floor beside head.**

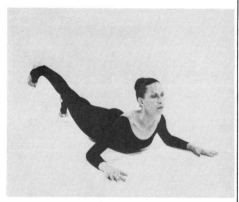

1 Lift head and R leg with flexed foot. Place ball of L foot on floor.
2-4 Push yourself up from floor and walk back on hands to L leg.

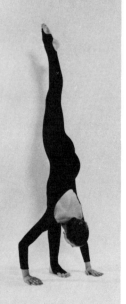

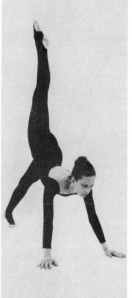

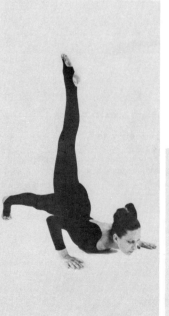

5-8 Stretch over L leg.

1-7 Walk forward on hands with R leg lifted all the time.

8 Return to START.

Repeat from the beginning several times, alternating sides.

44. Chest Lift

Another exercise which builds strength in the back, this one develops a good kick to the back, improves the attitude and arabesque to the back. When you lift your arms from the floor, be sure that your legs remain on the floor. Take your head as far as possible to aid in holding the position.—MM.

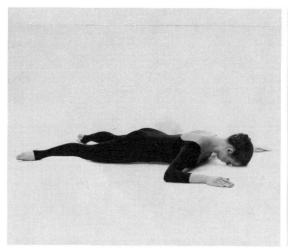

START by lying on stomach with legs turned out, slightly apart, hands on floor next to head.

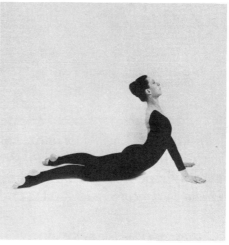

1-8 Lift head and chest and push back with hands to high arch.

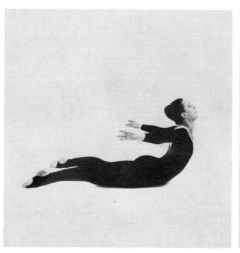

1 Stretch arms back, parallel to floor with palms out.
2-4 Hold and enlarge position.

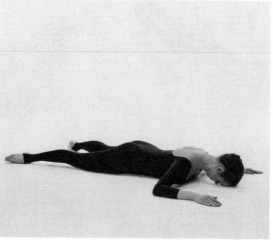

5-8 Lower chest and arms to starting position. Repeat from the beginning several times.

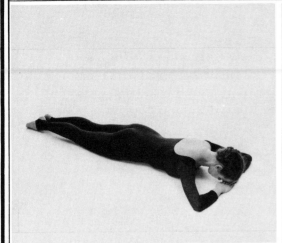

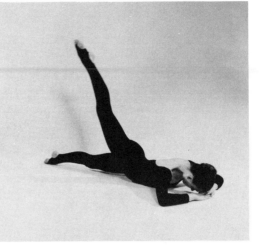

3-8 Repeat kick with L/R/L leg.

Repeat PART 1 several times.

START by lying on your stomach with legs in pp, hands under forehead.

PART 1:
1-2 Kick R leg up and put it down. Accent.

The Hip-Roll was designed for one reason: to aid the student who has a tendency to be a bit too heavy in the hips. It is good for the stomach as well. If you do it consistently every day, you can get very good results reducing the size of your hips and buttocks. It is also a usable movement in dance, as well.—MM.

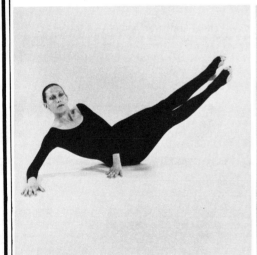

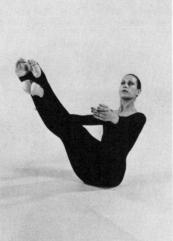

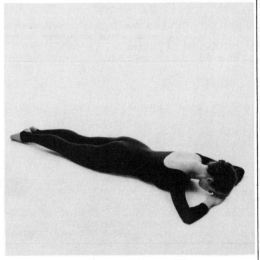

PART 2: Hip-Roll:
1 Lift chest and roll over to R hip, supporting yourself with arms on floor on R side of body. Lift legs parallel together and swing them to L.

2-3 Swing legs forward (above), R and back, while keeping body facing front. Stretch arms forward.

4 Return to starting position.

Repeat Hip-Roll several times, alternating sides.

The Long Stretch is also a usable movement in dance, but it has many other benefits. It builds strength in the arms and shoulders. It's a good exercise for opening up the hips and for working the back muscles from a straight-back position to the arched back (and back again). It is the preliminary exercise to the Pop-Up. When you do the Long Stretch, never take your eyes from the palm of the working hand. Try for the highest body arch that you can achieve—the longest possible curved line.

Practice the Long Stretch slowly in the beginning and then quickly, after you master the sequence. Do it with 8 counts up and down, then 4 counts up and down, and finally 2 counts up and 2 counts down.—MM.

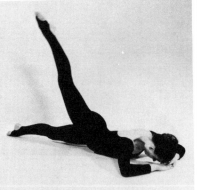

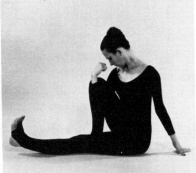

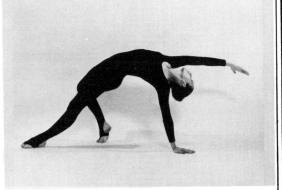

PART 3: Long Stretch
1-2 Kick R leg up (above). Roll to R and sit up facing pt 5, legs parallel, R foot flat on floor in to R hip. Sit on both hips and flex L

foot. Keep back straight, fold R arm, relax R hand and head. Support with L hand on floor behind L hip.

3-4 Lift R heel, causing L foot to point, as you push up and stretch R arm overhead parallel to floor, palm down. Look into R palm. Accent.

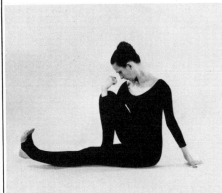

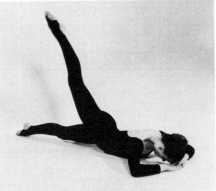

Repeat Long Stretch several times, alternating sides.

5-6 Sit down on both hips, as in center picture above.

7 Roll over to L hip. Stretch R leg parallel up behind. Point both feet. Place R hand back on floor.
8 Return leg to starting position (above).

In both the Long Stretch and the Pop-Up, keep your pelvis flat, parallel to the ceiling. In the long stretch, arch your back and rest your weight equally on the supporting hand, the ball of one foot, and the flat foot of the other leg.—MM.

In the Pop-Up, you need to make a quick return to standing position after going to the floor. If you use it correctly, you'll develop a quick and total body response from sitting to standing position. As with the Long Stretch, practice the Pop-Up slowly in the beginning, and then quickly, after you master it. Start by using 4 counts for each part of the exercise: 4 counts to lift the leg, 4 counts to make the Pop-Up, 4 counts to return to sitting position (leg in the air), and 4 counts to rest with the leg on the floor. After that, do it with 2 counts and finally with one count for each position. When you get the sequence technically correct, use it to go from sitting to standing position.

Remember to keep your body flat and rest your weight equally on the supporting hand and the balls of the feet while you practice the movement and push your weight forward into your thighs as you push yourself up to standing position.—MM.

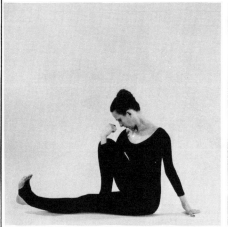

PART 4: Pop-Up
1-2 **Sit, facing pt 5, legs parallel, R foot flat on floor. Sit on both hips, flex L foot. Keep back straight. Fold R**

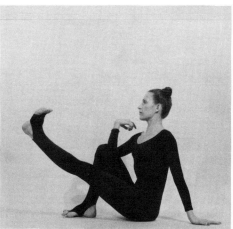

arm, relax hand and head. Support with **L hand on floor behind L hip.**
AND Lift L leg with flexed foot (above).

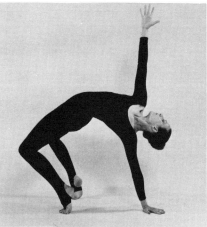

3 **Place L foot parallel to R in small 2p as you push pelvis up and stretch R arm to ceiling, palm in. Lift both heels.**
4 **Hold and enlarge position.**

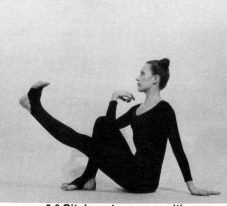

5-6 **Sit down to same position as center picture above.**

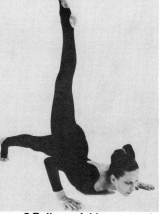

7 **Roll over L hip as you stretch R leg up parallel behind. Place R hand on floor for support.**
8 **Return to starting position.**

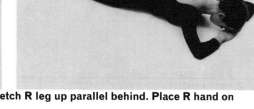

Repeat Pop-Up several times, alternating sides. The last time, use the Pop-Up as a quick recovery to standing position. Then turn to front and fall forward to stomach position (keep leg in air while falling), ready to start from the beginning to the other side.—MM.

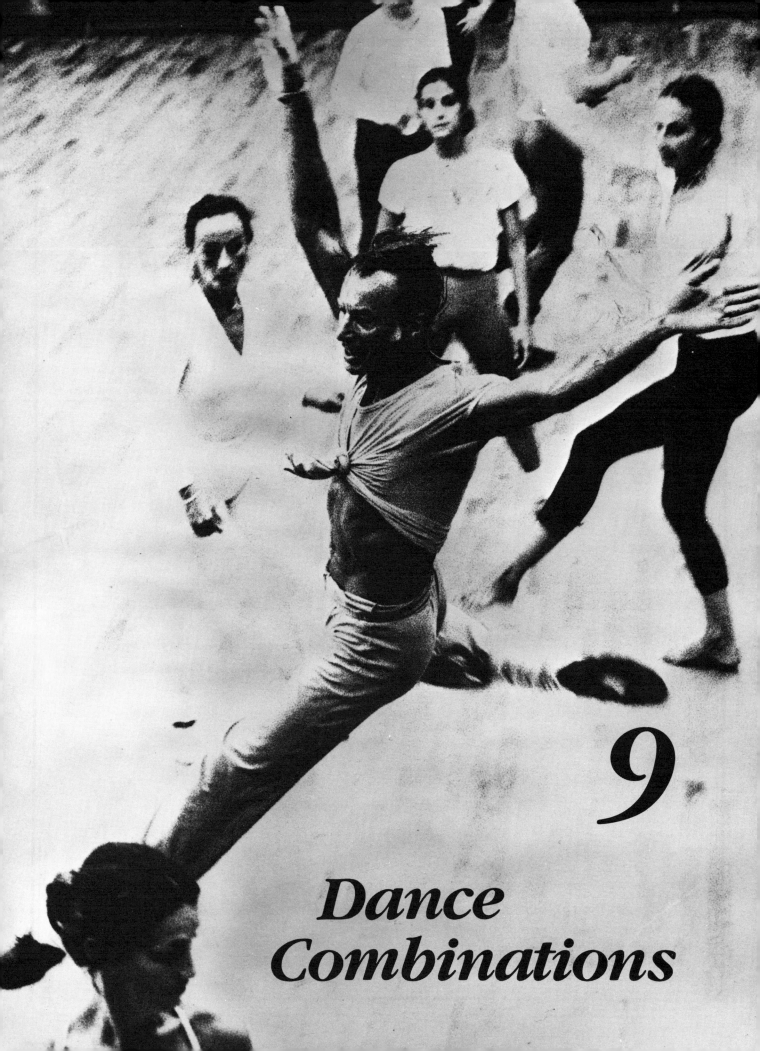

9

Dance Combinations

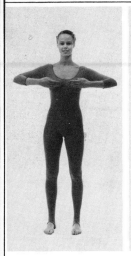 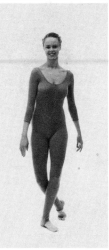 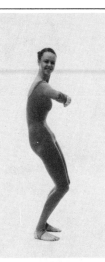 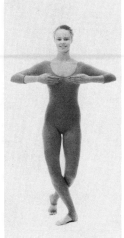 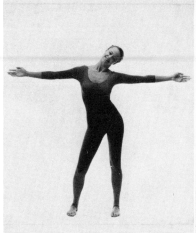

START in 1pp, arms in 1p.

AND 1 Ball-change R leg under, letting arms fall.

2-3 Close R leg in 1pp demi-plié to pt 7, contracting hard forward. Arms to 1p. Accent.

4 Step R leg over L to pt 1.

5 Place L leg slightly bent to side on flat foot. Lift L hip up, tilt head to L, take arms to 2p. Accent.

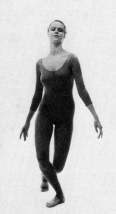 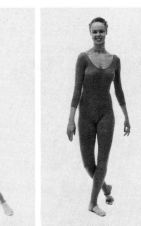 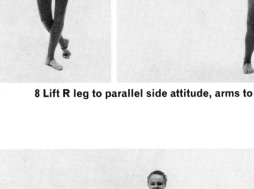

6 AND 7 Pas de bourré sideways to pt 3. L leg under R, R to side, L over R, letting arms hang naturally.

8 Lift R leg to parallel side attitude, arms to 3p middle, R in front.

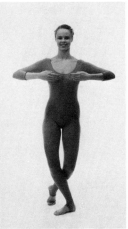 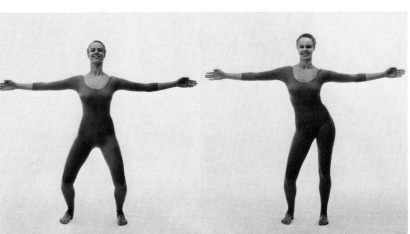 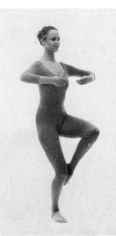

1 Step R leg over L, arms to 1p.

2-3 Place L leg in small 2 pp demi-plié and make half figure 8 with L hip. Arms to 2p. Soft movement forward, L and back.

4 Lift L leg to passé parallel facing pt 8. Arms to 1p.

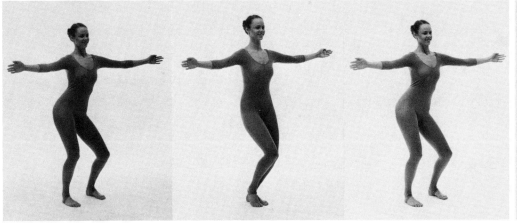

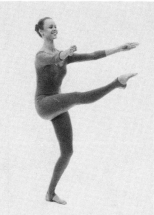

5 AND 6 Step L, R, L sideways to pt 6 (2p, 1p, 2p, letting hips move slightly R/L/R). Arms to 2p.

AND 7 Lift R leg straight forward, parallel to floor. Let arms fall; then lift them parallel to legs, palms in.

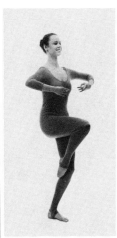

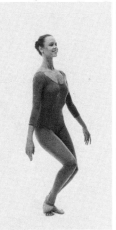

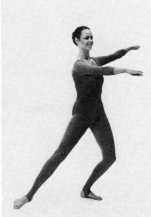

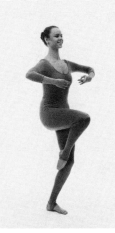

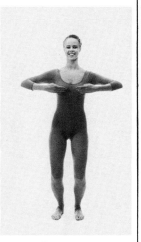

AND R leg to passé parallel, arms to 1p.

8 Lower R foot to ball in 1pp demi-plié, without weight.

1 R leg to side, relaxed, arms in 3p.

2-3 Quickly open arms to 2p and pull them into 1p as you do en dehors turns on L leg with R leg in passé parallel.

AND Close R leg in 1p, facing pt 1.

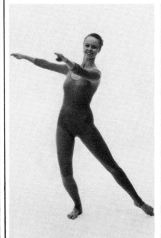

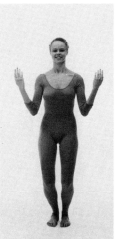

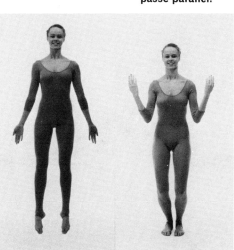

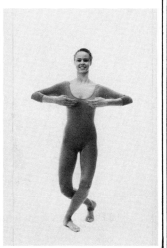

4 Place L leg to side relaxed. Arms to 3p middle.

5 Close L leg in 1pp, fold arms.

AND 6 Jump and land in 1pp, taking arms down, palms forward as you jump, and folding them as you land.

7 Step L leg over R with arms in 1p.

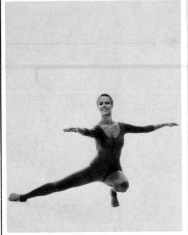

8-1 Grand plié on L leg with R leg relaxed to side. Keep weight in L thigh, arms to 3p middle. Straight back. Bounce back up like a ball.

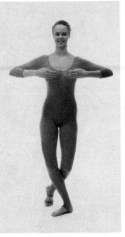

2 Step R leg over L, arms in 1p.

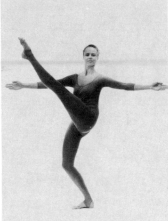

3 Flick L leg, crossed to R diagonal forward, arms in 2p.

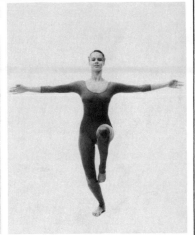

AND L leg to passé parallel.

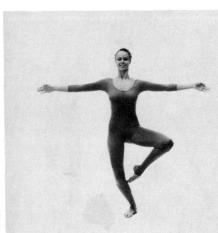

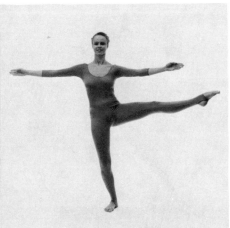

4 Flick L leg open to side, leaving it out.

5 Step L leg to pt 7.

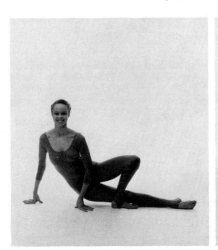

6 Bend L leg completely with R stretched under. Support yourself with hands on floor in front of you.

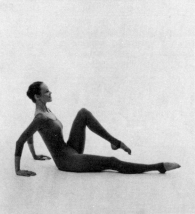

7-1 Sit on R hip and swing straight legs up to ceiling, one at a time, sitting on both hips.

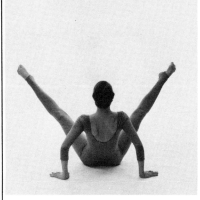

Support yourself with hands behind hips.

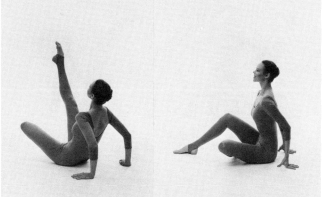

2 Bend L leg on floor (outside of leg touching floor) and place R leg bent over L with flat foot on floor. Arms support behind hips.

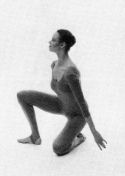

3 Use hands to push yourself off floor and step up on R leg.

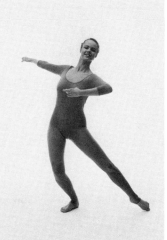

Place L leg to side relaxed, R arm to 2p, palm down, L arm to 1p. Face pt 1.

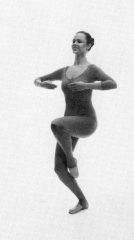

4-5 Quickly open L arm and close it in 1p with R arm as you turn en dehors on R leg with L in passé parallel.

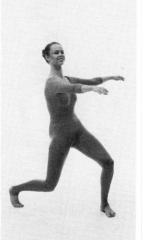

AND 6 Step out of turn by ball-change L/R to 4p, turned in (L forward), arms in 3p middle.

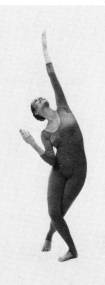

7 Step R leg over L. Fold R arm and stretch L up through 1p. Contract R side (face pt 1).
8 Hold and enlarge position.

47. Dance Combination B—Kari Helgesen

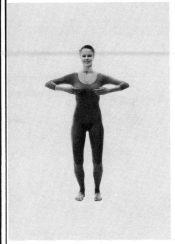 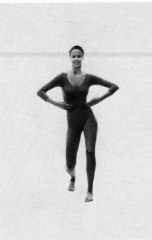 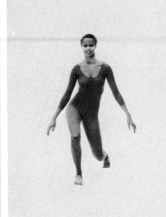 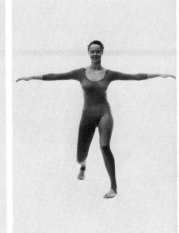

START in 1pp, demi-plié, with arms in 1p.

1-3 Step R/L/R leg back, pushing pelvis L/R/L, taking arms down and to 2p. Finish with palms down. All this in soft movements.

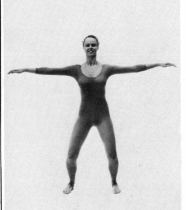 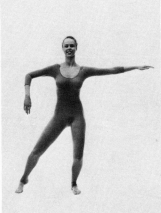 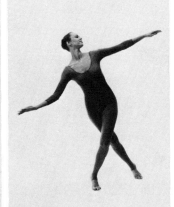 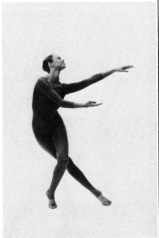

4-5 Step L leg to pt 7. Place R leg straight under on outside of foot. Go up on ball of L foot. Contract L side and make 1 outward circle with R arm, finishing by stretching it to L, palm up. Accent.

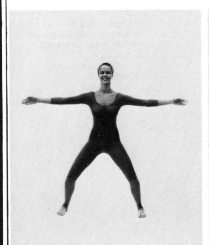 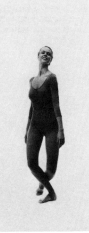 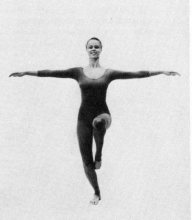 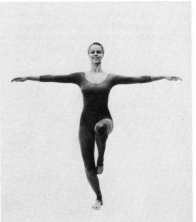

6 Step R leg to pt 3, swinging R arm down and to 2p.

AND 7 Ball-change L under R (let arms hang naturally).

8 AND Hip-fall to L with arms in 2p, palms down: Lift L leg to passé parallel. Lift L hip on bent R leg, lift R heel.

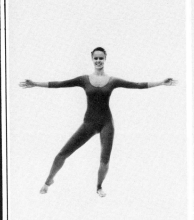
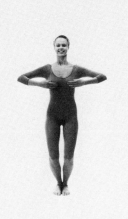
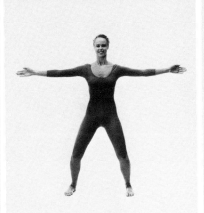
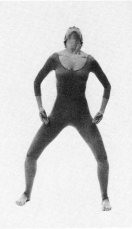

Step **L** to pt 7, leaving **R** leg to side. **Soft movement.**

1 Close R leg in 1pp, demi-plié and arms in 1p.

2 Slide out to 2pp with arms in 2p.

3 Release down, hitting yourself at break of hips with outsides of stiff hands.

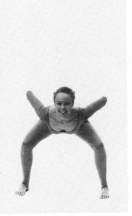
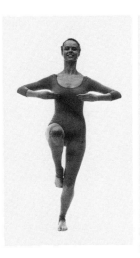
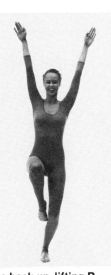
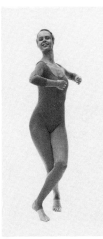
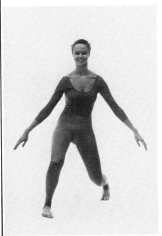

Breathe out. Finish with head down. Accent!

4 Breathe in as you come back up, lifting **R** leg to passé parallel. Stretch arms up through 1p.

5 Fold arms. Stretch them diagonally forward and down, palms down

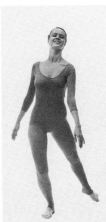

as you place **R** leg forward to 4p, turned out.

6 Rond de jambe á terre en dedans with **L** leg, letting arms hang naturally. **Soft movement.**
7 Finish with **L** leg forward and pull it over **R**, both heels lifted, equal weight, twisting upper body to **L**. **Accent.**

8 L leg to side, relaxed, folding arms, twisting upper body to **R**. **R** foot flat. **Face pt 1.**

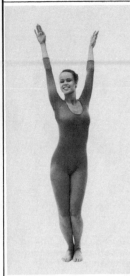

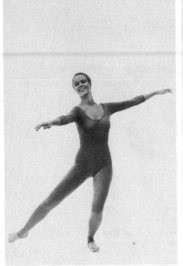

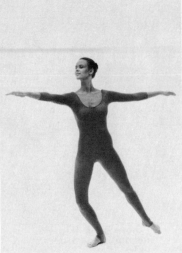

AND **Close L** leg in 1pp demi-plié. Stretch arms up.

1 Place R leg to side, relaxed, and open arms to 2p (palms down), twisting upper body to **L**.

2-3 **Step R** leg to pt 2 and turn on it en dedans with **L** leg stretched to side, down and turned out, just off floor. Arms in 2p, palms down.

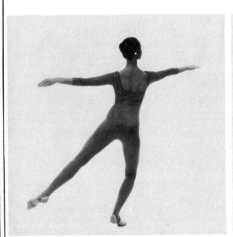

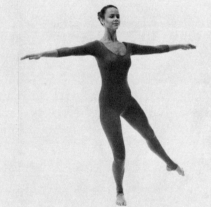

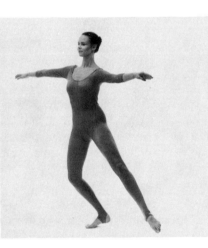

—(continuation of 2-3)—

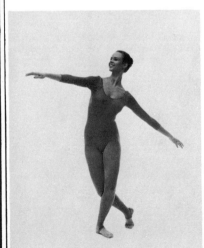

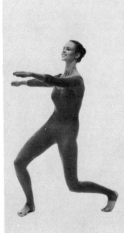

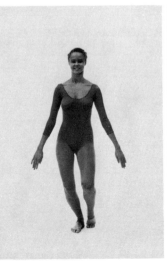

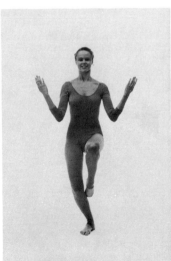

AND **4 Step L/R**/forward to pt 2 to 4p, turned in. Let **L** arm fall slightly down and forward to meet **R** arm in 3p middle.

5 Tap L foot on the ball in 1pp demi-plié, letting arms fall, palms back.

AND **Lift L** leg to passé parallel with accent. Fold arms.

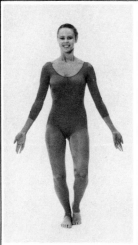 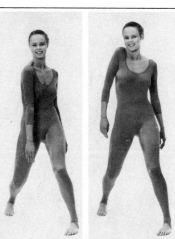 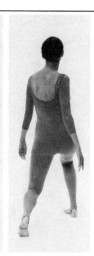

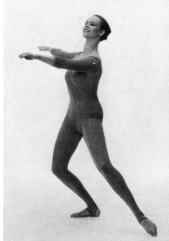

6 Lower L leg in 1pp, heel slightly off floor, letting arms fall, palms forward.

AND 7 Ball-change R, L to 4p, turned in, R foot back.
8 Shoulder-roll with R forward/up/back and change direction to pt 5, finishing in 4p, turned in, R leg in front.

1 Shoulder-roll L/forward/ up/back, changing direction back

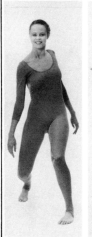 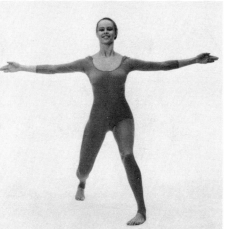 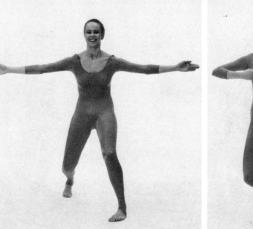 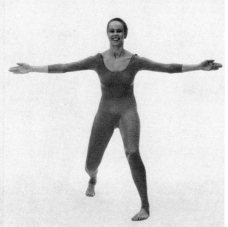

to pt 1.

2 Ripple with arms in 2p.

3 R leg under L, arms to 1p.

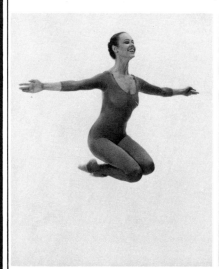 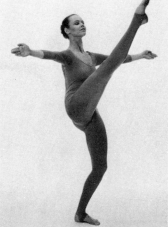 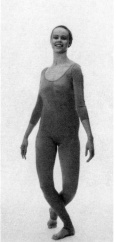 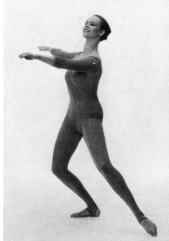

AND 4 Lift both legs underneath you and land on L leg, flicking R leg forward simultaneously. Arms to 2p. Face pt 8. Land on L leg.

AND 5 Step R leg over L and place L to side, relaxed, twisting upper body to R. Let arms fall and take them to 3p middle. Finish facing pt 2.

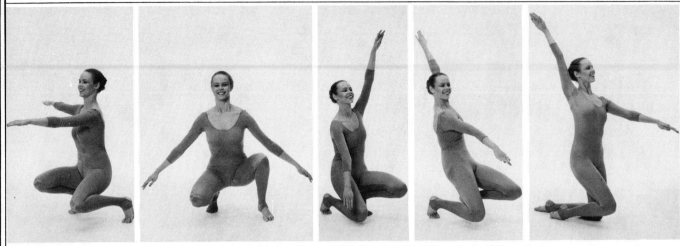

6-8 Sit in grand plié, keeping weight in both thighs. Change direction to pt 8, R knee just off floor. Swing arms down and forward as you "walk through" positions of legs, swinging L arm, then R forward, up, back (windmill arms) to help you come off the floor.

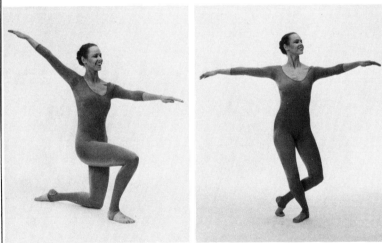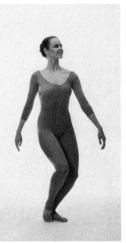

Step up on R leg over L. Arms in 2p, palms down twisting body to R.

1 Take weight back on L leg and place R leg back to 4p, turned in (passing through 1pp). Let arms swing down and to 3p middle, with R in front.

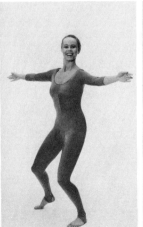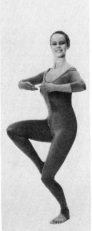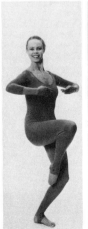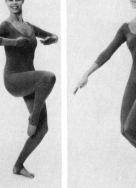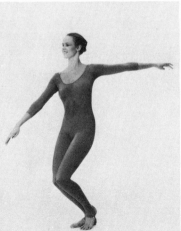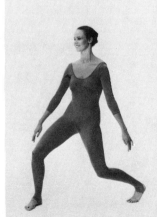

2 Open the position of the feet to the R and turn on L leg en dehors with R leg in passé parallel. Arms to 1p.

AND 3-4 Close R leg in 1p demi-plié facing pt 2. Place L leg back to 4p, turned in, R arm low, L arm back.

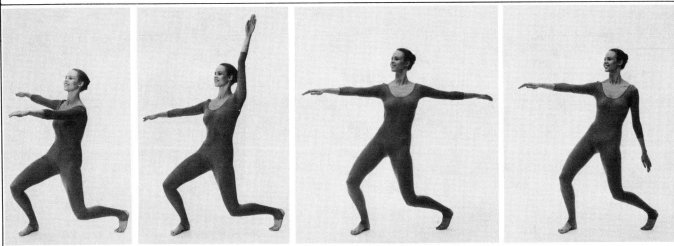

Swing a straight **L** arm from the shoulder forward/up/back 1¾ times, finishing up with accent as you lift **L** leg to passé parallel with **R** leg on half-toe. **R** arm forward, palm down.

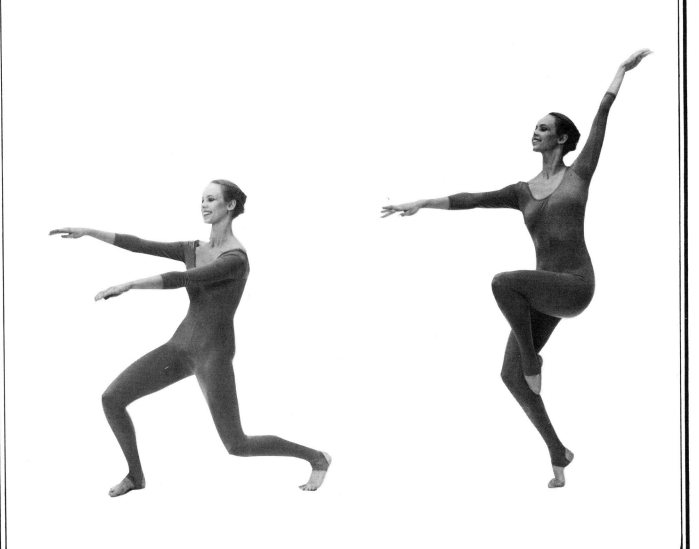

48. Dance Combination C—Matt Mattox

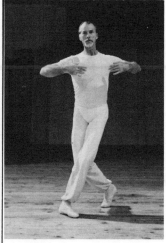
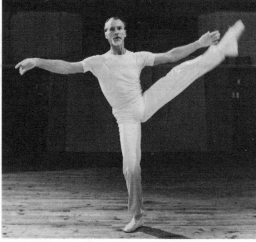
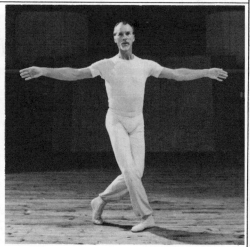

START in 1pp, arms down.
1 Step R leg under L, both slightly out. Arms to 1p.

2 Flick L leg to side, turned out. Arms to 2p.

3 Step L leg under R, both slightly out.

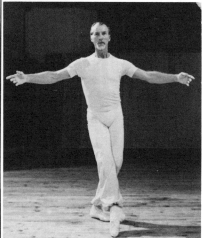
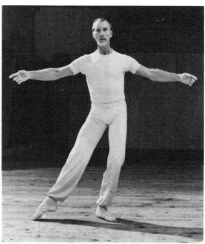
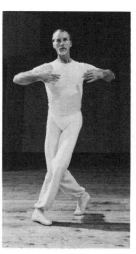
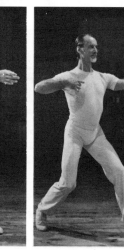

4 R leg rond de jambe á terre en dehors.

5 Finish rond de jambe with R leg under L and arms in 1pp.

6 Step R over L, letting arms fall.

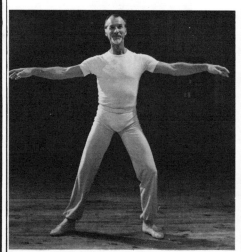
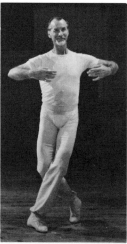

7 AND 8 Step L/R/L to pt 8 (R leg under L), lifting arms to 2p. Finish by closing R arm in 1p with feet in 4p turned in, L foot in front.

AND Stretch R arm diagonally L forward at shoulder level. Contract slightly forward. L arm to 1p.

1 R arm to 1p. L arm to 2p and release.

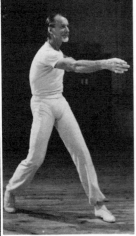
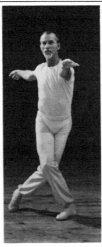
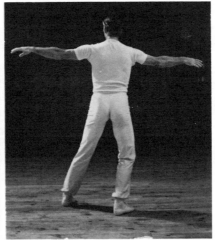
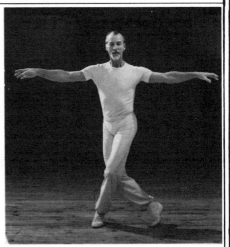

2 Stretch **R** arm diagonally forward at shoulder level. **Contract slightly forward. L** arm to 1p.

AND R arm to 1p. **3** Facing front, but twisting slightly to **R,**

place **L** leg under **R,** arms 2p. **4** Hold and enlarge position.

5–8 Unwind to **L,** leaving arms in 2p.

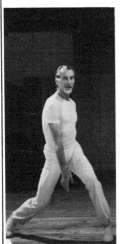
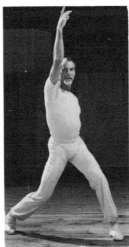
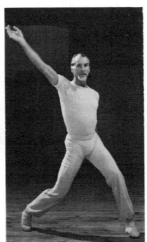
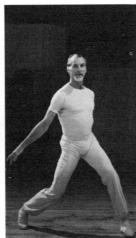
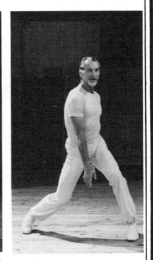

7 Place **R** leg back to 4p, turned in, facing pt 8. Swing **R** arm forward/overhead/back/down. **L** arm down.

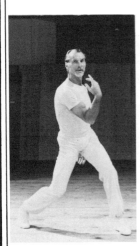
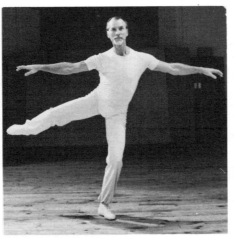
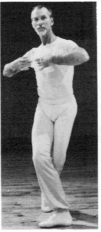
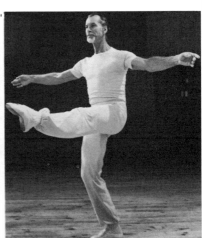

8 Contract forward and fold **R** arm.
1 Hold and enlarge position.

2 Facing front, lift **R** leg to attitude parallel to side. Arms to 2p.

3 Step **R** leg over **L.** Arms to 1p.

4 Flick **L** leg diagonally **R** forward. Take arms to 2p.

115

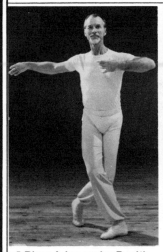
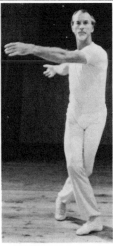
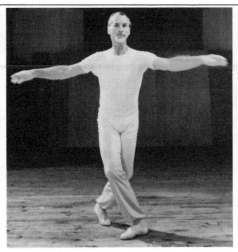
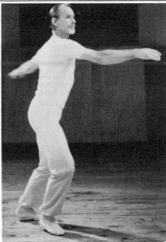

5 Place L leg under R with L arm in 1p.

AND Open L arm diagonally R forward.

6 Open legs and arms to 2p and turn en dehors on R leg—

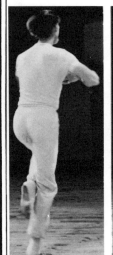
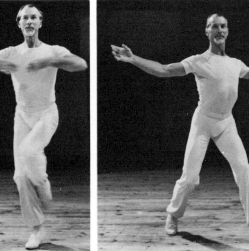
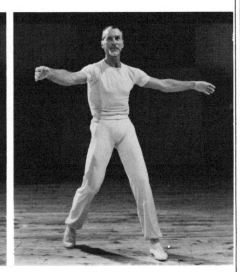

with L leg in passé parallel and arms in 1p.

AND 7 Place L leg in 1pp and R leg back to 4p turned in. Arms in 2p (to pt 8). AND 8 Release—

Contract—

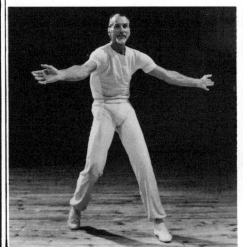
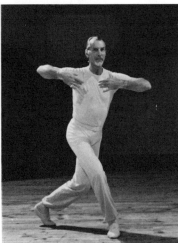
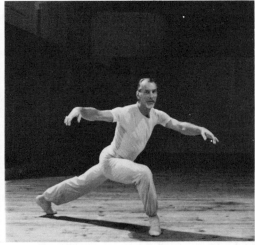

ribcage and hips.

1 Step L leg under R. Arms to 1p.

2 Stretch out L leg to a deep position on ball of L foot. Arms 3p middle.

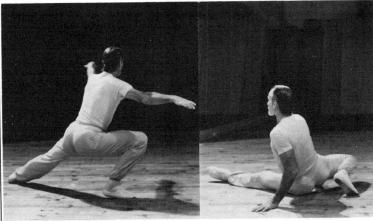

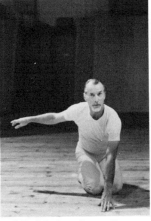

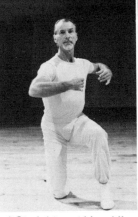

3-4 Turn out **L** leg, arms to 2p and sit on floor in 4p split, **L** leg straight in front. Support with arms on floor (to pt 4).

5 Pull in legs beneath you, facing front. Sit on heels. **R** arm in 2p. **L** arm supports on floor in front.

6 Straighten at hip while placing bent **L** leg forward on floor. Step on it. Arms 1p.

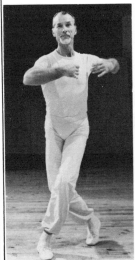

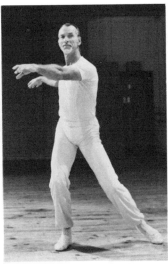

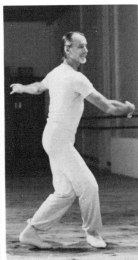

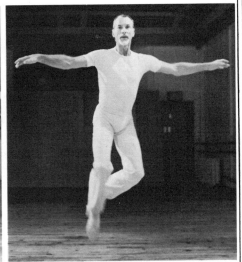

7 Step **R** leg under **L**.

8 Place **L** leg relaxed to side. Arms to 3p middle.

1 Put weight on **L** leg and step **R** leg over it. **R** arm halfway closing to 1p. **L** to 2p. (to pt 8).

AND Pull up **R** leg to passé turned out as you jump and fold **L** leg, slightly turned out in air. Arms in 2p,

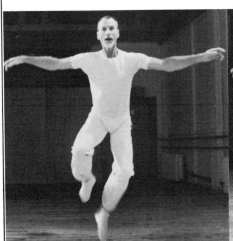

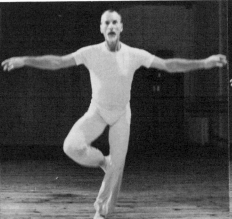

changing direction to front.

2 Land on **L** leg with **R** under **L**.

48. Dance Combination C—Matt Mattox (page 5)

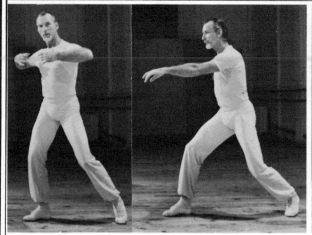

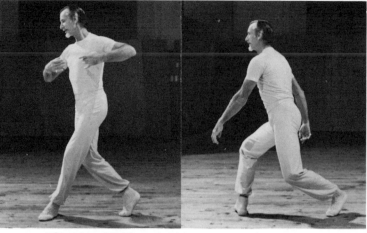

AND 3 Step L/R to 4p turned in (R in front), taking arms through 1p to 3p middle, and facing pt 2.

AND 4 Step L and R forward, taking arms through 1p and down (pt 3).

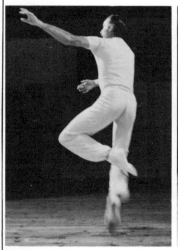

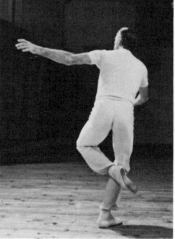

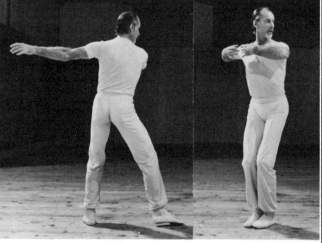

AND Pull up L leg to passé turned out as you fold R leg (slightly turned out in air) and jump sideways (to your left) facing back wall. R arm to 1p, L to 2p.

5-6 Land on R leg (above) and step L to 2p. Arms in 3p middle, R in front.

7 AND 8 Step R/L/R, turning to your R to pt 7 with arms and feet—2p—1p—

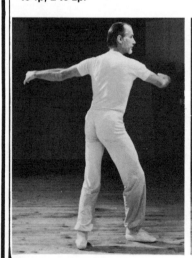

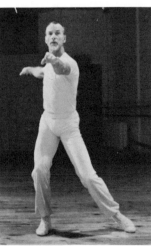

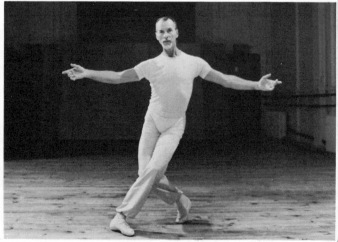

and 2p.

1 Finish turning by placing L leg, relaxed, to side. Twist upper body to R, facing front. Arms to 2p.

AND 2 Take weight onto L leg and step R leg in place (ball-change).
3 Step L leg over R and—

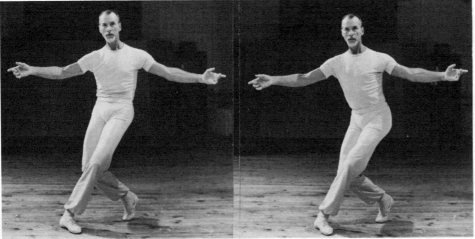

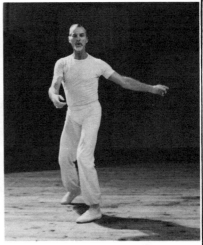

roll pelvis R/forward/L/back.

4-5 Place R leg back to 4p turned in and roll R shoulder

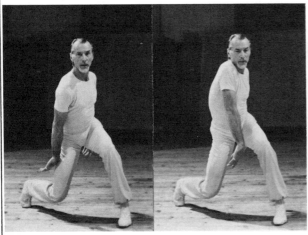

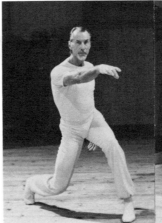

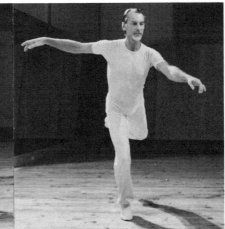

forward, up and back, L arm down (pt 8).

Finish with R arm lifted forward at shoulder level.

6 Take weight onto R leg and lift L leg to parallel back attitude. Arms in 3p middle.

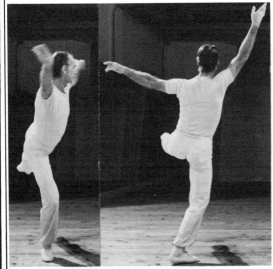

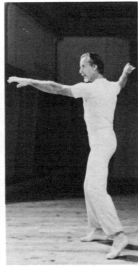

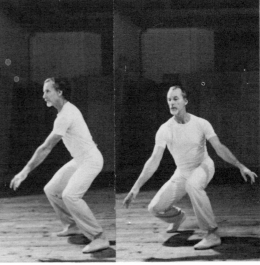

AND 7 Stretch L leg parallel to R diagonal back. Turn it out and change direction to pt 4, finishing with arms in 3p high.

AND Step L leg to pt 4. 8 Step R leg to pt 4, slightly turned in. Arms to 3p middle.

AND 1 Start 4p jump by going well into plié. Swing arms down and up to help you to jump diagonally L and forward with L leg in front.

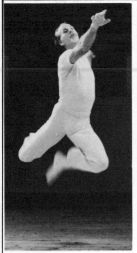

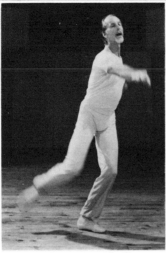

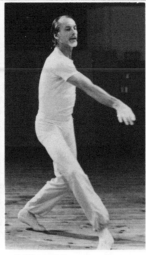

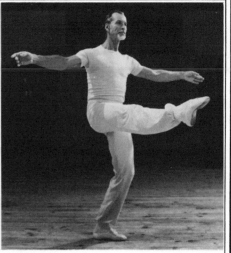

R arm finishes diagonally forward and up, L arm in 2p. Twist upper body to L. Look up at R hand.

2 Land on L leg (to pt 8).

3 Step R leg over L, taking R arm diagonally forward and down. L arm down.

4 Take weight back to L leg and flick R leg forward, with arms through 1p and 2p.

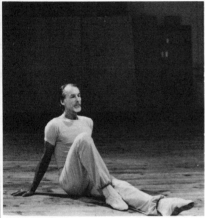

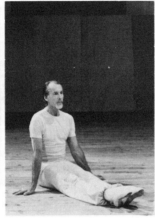

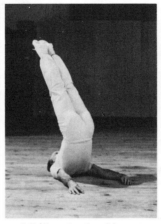

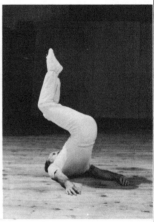

AND Step R leg back. 5 Bend R knee completely and sit on floor with L leg straight in front. Support with arms behind you.

AND Stretch R leg forward. Use arms to push yourself diagonally back.

6 Roll up to shoulder stand with parallel legs extended to ceiling.

7 Break at hip and knees. Turn knees to R as you roll down to your back.

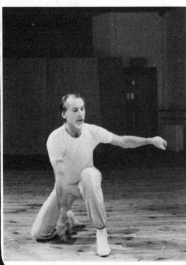

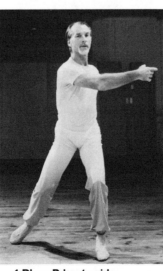

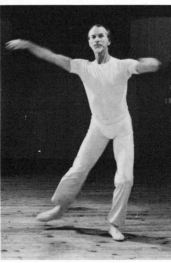

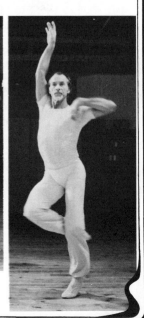

AND 8 Finish rolling down with bent R leg on floor and step up on L leg. Arms in 3p low.

1 Place R leg to side, relaxed, arms to 3p middle.

2 Turn en dehors on L leg, lifting R to passé parallel. Close L arm in 1p and swing R arm from 2p and overhead—

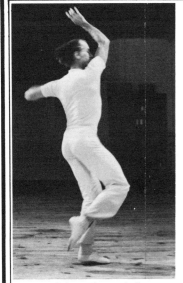

and down towards **L** arm.

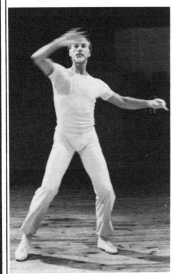

3 Facing front, step **R** leg to 2pp and finish with **R** arm bent in front of head/ forward/2p.

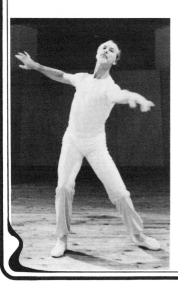

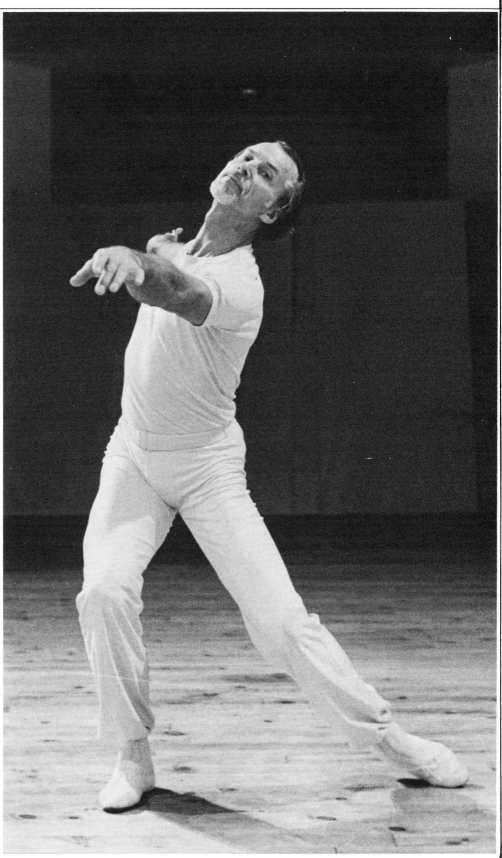

4 Finish combination with weight on **R** leg, **L** leg to side relaxed. Arms in 2p, twisting upper body to **R**.

Glossary

Accent—With attack.

Attitude—A lift of the leg from the hip with a bent knee—forward, side or back—parallel or turned out.

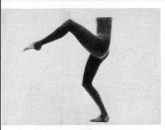

Forward parallel: the knee points up.

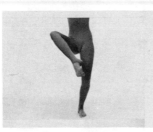

Forward turned out: knee points to side.

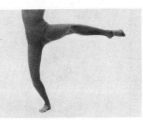

Side attitude parallel: knee points forward.

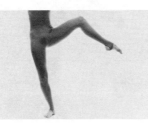

Side attitude turned out: knee points up.

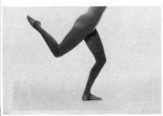

Back attitude parallel: knee points down.

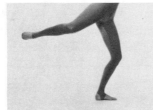

Back attitude turned out: knee points to side.

Ball-change—A change in balance from ball of one foot to flat or ball of the other foot. Direction and pattern as desired.

Circle of the arm—A bend from the elbow with the lower arm in a circle that starts and finishes in 2p. The upper arm is kept skill.

INWARD CIRCLE

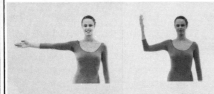

START with half circle up—go on to 1p.

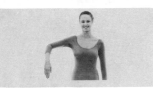

Make half-circle down—and back to 2p.

The outward circle goes down first, and to 1p; then it circles up and back to 2p.

Contraction—

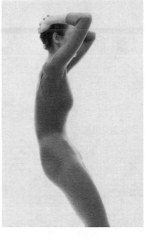

Matt's definition:
"The gathering together of any muscle or group of muscles, from a relaxed position to a hard conditioned muscle. Typical is the bicep. Relaxed, the muscle is long and soft. Contracted it becomes bulgy, round and hard." This term is often applied to the reduction in size between the ribcage and pelvis. Ribcage is pushed back, pelvis forward.

En croix—In a cross (forward/side/back/side).

En dedans—Inward (for some movements it means circling in toward body).

En dehors—Outward (for some movements it means circling away from the body).

Enlarge—To keep the energy flowing in a position, not just to hold it.

Flick—A kick where the leg is bent through passé on the way out, and generally on the way in. The foot is usually pointed (but may be flexed). The standing leg is always bent in this style. A flick may be done in all directions and at all levels.

Flip hand—A relaxed hand that strikes out, in, up or down. In this style, it is used mostly as the arm opens from 1p to 2p.

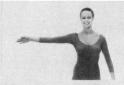

Open lower arm halfway (palm relaxed inwards) and send out hand with force as you stretch arm. Stop movement just before elbow is stretched completely.

Folded arm—Arm bent in front of chest, elbow down, palm in. Open lower arm slightly.

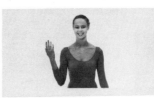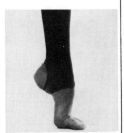

Half-toe—To ball of foot.

Hip-Push—A contraction of waist and buttocks muscles in a long and soft movement in any direction. To the back, buttocks muscles are released.

Kick—A straight-knee kick, foot pointed or flexed, in any direction and at any level. Standing leg is always bent in this style.

Lifted heel—A lift of the heel above the floor, adjusted to your own balance.

Over and Under—When stepping *over*, one leg is crossed in front of the other. When placing one leg *under*, one leg is crossed behind the other. In both cases, the front leg has the weight and back heel is lifted. Both legs are naturally turned out. Upper body is slightly twisted in opposition to the lower body when used in combinations. Done rapidly, the legs cross over more so that thighs touch each other.

See pictures under *Pas de Bourré*: picture at L shows R leg *under* L leg; picture at R shows R leg *over* L leg.

Parallel Side Attitude—see *Attitude*.

Pas de Bourré—In this context, stepping sideways or turning—under, side, over—keeping knees bent. In pictures below, you see:

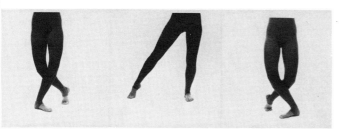

R leg under L—L leg to side—R leg over.

Passé—A movement of the leg through a position where the foot is pointed along the inside of the knee of the standing leg. Standing leg can be bent or straight.

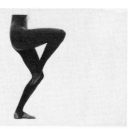 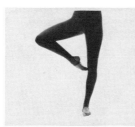

When knee of working leg points forward, it is passé parallel (above). When big toe points

along inside of the knee, and knee of working leg is to the side, it is passé turned out.

Plié—A knee-bend with *resistance*, keeping knees over toes and equal weight in a parallel or turned-out position.

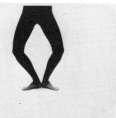 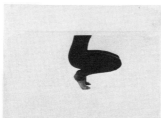

Demi-plié: half, with heels on floor (here in 1p, turned out).

Grand plié: full, heels off floor, passing through demi-plié on the way down and up (here in 1pp).

Positions—See pages 11 and 12 for photographs of arm and leg positions as well as positions on the floor.

Relaxed leg forward—

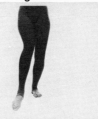

Leg slightly turned in and bent, with outside of big toe on floor, without weight.

Relaxed leg to the side—

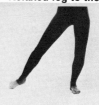

Leg parallel, slightly bent. Heel lifted, outside of big toe on floor, without weight. (When lifted in this position, leg is in side attitude parallel.)

Release—

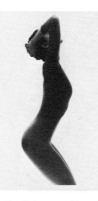

Matt's definition:
"The opposite of the contraction. If the muscles are brought into a contracted condition, the release is the *de-contract* that relaxes the muscles." The term is often applied to the disengagement where the ribcage is pushed forward and the pelvis back.

Resistance—Dancing as if you were in water. It means you must put more muscle power into the slow, smooth movement than when you're surrounded by air only.

Ripple—A continuous release/contract movement through ribcage and pelvis: release vertebra by vertebra from the bottom of spine up to head, then contract in same way.

Rond de Jambe—A circular movement of the leg, it circles into or away from the body: *par terre*: on the floor
en l'air: in the air

Shimmy—A shoulder-shake, where one shoulder is pushed forward and the other back simultaneously in very quick tempo.

Tendu—A slide of the working foot (parallel or turned out, forward, side or back) with straight knee. The foot glides along the floor through 2p or 4p to the utmost point possible, with big toe on the floor and heel lifted. In this context, the foot starts in and returns to 1p. Here you see it with parallel feet.

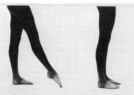

Under—See Over and Under.

Unwind—Starting with L leg over R, for example: Turn to R (leaving feet on floor with heels slightly lifted), staying in plié. Come around to the other side, finishing with R leg over L.

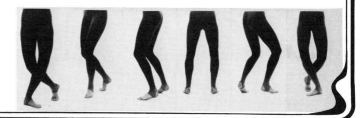

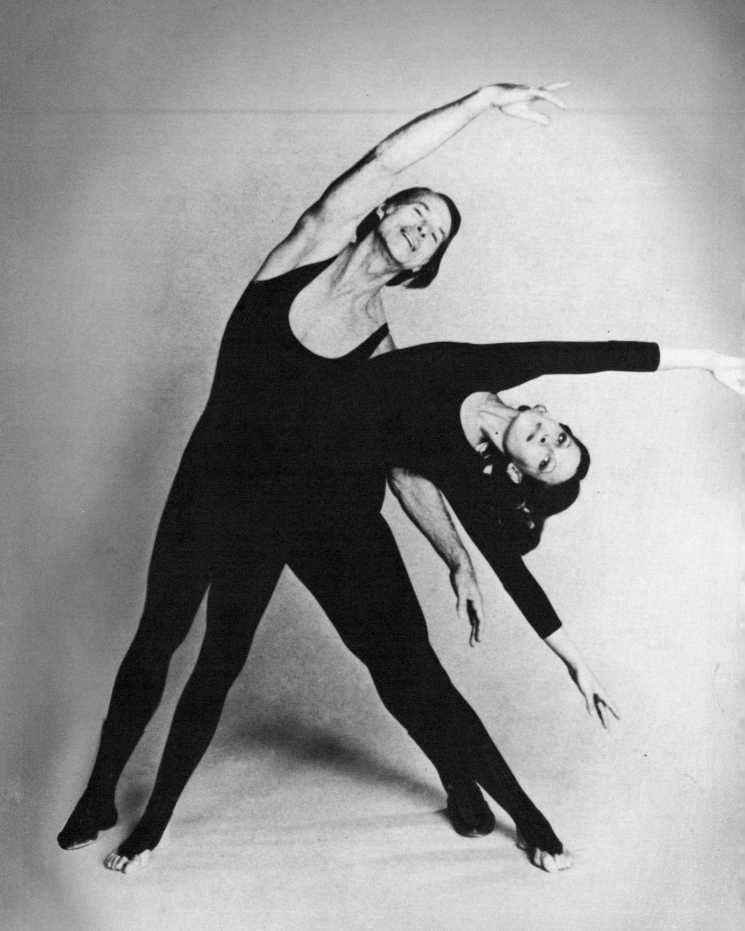

Afterword by Matt Mattox

In the beginning, I developed this system of dance in order to teach the professional dancer how to use isolation—isolation of the different parts of the body. Then in time, as I worked more with beginners, I realized that the key to this form of dance lies in a mental change. When the student realizes that coordination of the body begins with the brain and then extends to the body, he or she arrives at an understanding of what dance—of any kind—is all about.

For the beginner, work on the isolations—mental and physical—is relatively simple. But for the student who wants to be a professional dancer, the mental and physical work becomes more difficult and complicated, and it is vitally important. Through the isolations, the student trains the mind; these mental processes result in physical sensations through which the individual becomes more and more aware and interested in the workings of his or her own body.

It is the complicated isolation exercises that bring all of this into being. That's why arm work has been added to the simple isolations provided here. The use of any one part of the body is not so difficult, but when you add arm work to it—and head work to that—the technical aspects become complex—demanding great amounts of concentration and practice. As they are mastered, the reflexes become sharper and more in tune with the body.

As the student progresses in using isolations, it becomes increasingly important to translate the exercises into dance form—to realize that dance comes out of the exercises and to learn how to bring it out. The moment that this realization takes place, the dancer is born, and from this point on, the progress to perfection in this technique is only a matter of time.

Anyone can learn to dance. How well you learn depends on you—your will, your dedication, your love of dance.

Biography—Matt Mattox

Born in 1921 in Tulsa, Oklahoma, Matt Mattox began his career singing and dancing in an amateur children's program at the Fox Figueroa Theatre in California at age 11. Two months after that he was studying tap with Terry Kerr and then later with Evelyn Burns, who also introduced him to exhibition ballroom. By the time he was 16 he realized that all he wanted to do was dance, and he began studying classical dance with Lester Lane and Ernest Belcher.

In 1942 at the start of World War II, he enlisted as a glider pilot, later joining the regular U.S. Air Force as a fighter pilot for 22 months, flying P47 Thunderbolts.

In 1944 when he returned to California, Cyd Charisse got him an audition for MGM contract dancer; he signed a contract the same day. His first film, choreographed by Eugene Loring, was *Yolanda and the Thief* with Fred Astaire, and he also appeared in *Easy to Wed* with Lucille Ball and *Two Sisters from Boston* with June Allyson and Kathryn Grayson, both choreographed by Jack Donahue.

In 1946 he left MGM to work for Columbia Studios in New York with Jack Cole, who many say was the father of American jazz dance. Mattox' technique is strongly influenced by Cole's style and inspiration. While in New York, Mattox appeared in the musical comedy *Are You With It?* and in a play with music called *Park Avenue*. During the next years he made such films as *The Merry Widow* (with Cole) and *Walking My Baby Back Home*. He worked with Vera Zorina at the Civic Light Opera Association and then toured, as premier danseur in *Song of Norway*, with Alexandra Denisova (Patricia Denise).

In 1949 he went to Australia to play the dancing role of Curly in *Oklahoma!* for over two years.

Back in the U.S. in the early 50's he began working with Jack Cole steadily, doing such films as *The I Don't Care Girl* starring Mitzi Gaynor, and *There's No Business Like Show Business* and *Gentlemen Prefer Blondes* with Marilyn Monroe. He worked with Cole in the Broadway show *Carnival in Flanders*, in which he danced the flamenco and created a critical stir which won him the acting/singing/dancing part of eldest brother Caleb in *Seven Brides for Seven Brothers* (choreographed by Michael Kidd). He also appeared in *The Bandwagon*, choreographed by Michael Kidd and starring Fred Astaire and Cyd Charisse.

He sang and danced in the Broadway musical *The Vamp* with Carol Channing, appeared in the *Ziegfeld Follies of 1956* (with Cole), and again attracted major critical attention with his performance in the film *Pepe*, starring Cantinflas.

He began to do more choreography, creating the dances for the films *Hot Blood* with Jane Russell and *Glory Brigade*, as well as for a revival of *Annie Get Your Gun*. He choreographed other shows as well, including the Broadway production of Jules Styne's *Say Darling*. And he regularly choreographed all the dances on the prestigious television program The Bell Telephone Hour.

During the past years he had been teaching continuously: at the Eugene Loring School, at Showcase Studios, at the June Taylor School of Dance, for Rebecca Harkness, and finally, in 1958 at his own school.

In 1963 he taught in Europe for the first time at a summer course in Denmark. And shortly afterward, in 1964 he decided to leave the commercial theatre completely. He closed his own school and during the next years worked for New York University, the Neighborhood Playhouse, Morelli and other institutions.

It wasn't until 1970 that he taught in Norway for the first time, changing his form of teaching totally and developing the system that he uses today. He moved to London to teach at the Dance Centre, as well as at The Place, home of the London Contemporary Dance Theatre. He took several months off to tour Europe, teaching in Finland, Norway, Germany, Sweden and France as well as the U.S. While in Salt Lake City, he created the ballet "Jazz Opus Back" for the Repertory Dance Theatre.

In 1972 he created a workshop group which performed in Colombes, Paris, at the Edinburgh Festival and at the Round House in London, and in 1974 he started doing choreography for French television. In 1975 he moved to Paris to teach at the *Maison des Jeunes et de la Culture* (MJC) in Colombes.

Mattox continues to visit many European countries regularly, choreographing for professional dance companies as well as amateur groups, creating new ballets which have been receiving awards throughout Europe. In 1979 he opened his own school in Paris and moved it, in 1982, to Perpignan on the south coast of France. He teaches there and throughout Europe at seminars.

Biography—Elisabeth Frich

Born and educated in Oslo, Norway, Elisabeth Frich studied at Den Norske Balletthøyskole, a full-time school of dance which offers university degrees to dancers, teachers and choreographers. There she studied classical, modern and jazz dance, character dance, tap, ethnic dance and mime, as well as other related courses. She went on to train for two years in London with Matt Mattox at the Dance Center, where she also studied tap with Gillian Gregory, Graham technique with Robert Cohan, Jane Dudley, Irene Dilks and others; classical ballet with Anna Northcote and body conditioning with Alan Herdman.

She has performed with the Høvik Ballett, Jorunn Kirkenær's dance group, and with Matt Mattox' company, on stage and on many television programs.

She taught at the Dance Center in London, as assistant to Matt Mattox, and on her return to Oslo at Den Norske Balletthøyskole and the Norwegian Opera Ballet School. She has also taught special courses in jazz at the Norwegian University of Sports, at summer courses for the Finnish Dance Association, in Sweden at a seminar for the Nordic Theatre Committee, in Copenhagen at seminars, and in the U.S. at Ballet Binghamton (Master Classes in Mattox' technique).

She has choreographed fashion shows, numbers for television, and variety theatre shows in Norway.

A co-director and member of the board of Den Norske Balletthøyskole, she is also the director of her own Jazz Art Productions, dedicated to the promotion of Mattox' "Jazz Art Technique" and jazz dance in general. It is through that company that she produced the video cassette that shows all the exercises in this book (see page 10). The videotape was shown at the International Dance Film and Videotape Festival at Lincoln Center in New York in 1981.

Index